T0151689

PRAISE FOR *HEART TO BEAT*

"Brian Lima's story is a truly inspiring one. It is one of true heart—yes, of that remarkable indispensable part of our bodies, but even more so of the qualities of a man who grew to master surgery on it."

—ROALD HOFFMANN, PH.D.,
Frank H. T. Rhodes Professor of
Humane Letters at Cornell University;
Winner of the Nobel Prize in Chemistry, 1981;
author, *The Same and Not the Same*

"Brian has clearly articulated the personal character qualities that are the essential elements of every strong personal brand. This inspiring story is a good reminder that admired personal brands are powered by an authentic soul, dedicated to making a difference, not just a superficial image created through the buzz of social media."

—KARL D. SPEAK, best-selling author of
Be Your Own Brand

My friend and colleague, heart surgeon Dr. Brian Lima, one of the most committed and hardest working doctors I know, has written a compelling, rags-to-riches motivational manifesto for achieving professional fulfillment. Read it to learn the life philosophy of one of America's best young surgeons, and use it to realize your own goals."

—SANDEEP JAUHAR, *New York Times*
bestselling author of *Heart: A History*

"*Heart to Beat* is a personal tale of GRIT, of passion and perseverance, and will undoubtedly serve to inspire all those that wish to achieve top flight, just as Lima has accomplished in his journey—a lesson in attaining brilliance in professional pursuit while ensuring meaningfulness by a relentless focus on a value-driven life. The teachings and quotes in this captivating memoir will endure through their simple wisdom and serve to galvanize us all."

—MANDEEP R. MEHRA, MD, MSc, FRCP(London)
The William Harvey Distinguished Chair
in Advanced Cardiovascular Medicine
Executive Director, Center for Advanced Heart Disease,
Brigham and Women's Hospital
Professor of Medicine, Harvard Medical School
Editor-in-Chief, *The Journal of Heart
and Lung Transplantation*

"An inspiring story of triumph in the face of adversity. Against all odds, Dr. Lima succeeded and became a leading heart surgeon. In *Heart to Beat* he shares the strategies that can help all of us to succeed in our own lives."

—MARC GILLINOV, MD
Chair, Department of Thoracic &
Cardiovascular Surgery, Cleveland Clinic

"Lima deftly blends a useful guide with an absorbing autobiography; he doesn't concentrate excessively on either one.... Helpful advice from a keen, assertive, and relatable physician."

—Kirkus Reviews

In *Heart to Beat,* "heart transplant surgeon Lima, the child of Cuban immigrants to the U.S., turns his talents to self-help... an encouraging work intended to inspire readers to overcome mediocrity and live their best lives."

—BookLife Reviews

"*Heart to Beat* is a must read for anyone looking for a boost of confidence and inspiration to reach their full potential. Dr. Lima's story of hard-earned success is proof that sky's the limit when you're willing to put in the time and effort towards fulfilling your dreams."

—ELENA RIOS, MD, MSPH, FACP
President & CEO of National
Hispanic Medical Association

"Brian Lima's inspiring memoir *Heart to Beat* is about how he became a top heart surgeon...Steady in its pace, the text focuses on, and resolves, the challenges at each stage of Lima's life before it progresses. Each stage proved harder than the last, but Lima records exceptional accomplishments at each. Accessible discussions punctuate the chapters, pronouncing what should be learned from them and emphasizing relevant qualities to cultivate, like focus. The text ends in a hopeful way, though with the reminder that achieving dreams comes at a cost."

—Foreword Clarion Review

"*Heart to Beat* is like a great kitchen table chat with an old friend. It's a decent way to spend a few hours and perhaps rekindle your own passions and zeal for life."

— San Francisco Book Review, 5/5 Star Rating

HEART TO
BEAT

A cardiac surgeon's inspiring story of success
and overcoming adversity—*The Heart Way.*

BRIAN LIMA, M.D.

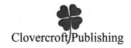

Clovercroft Publishing

Heart to Beat

Published by Clovercroft Publishing, Franklin, Tennessee

Image of the HeartMate 3™ Left Ventricular Assist System (LVAS) used by permission of Abbott Laboratories.

Edited by OnFire Books

Copy Edit by Lee Titus Elliott

Cover Design by Nelly Sanchez

Interior Design by Suzanne Lawing

Printed in the United States of America

978-1-950892-35-8

Dedication

To my amazing parents, Apolonio and Ramona, who selflessly and courageously fled Cuba in 1968, all for the hope of a better life for their family in the United States. I will always cherish your memory and the most valuable lesson you imparted to me, that a strong work ethic is the ultimate "talent"! To my beloved sister, Diana, whom I miss dearly, may you rest in peace. To my amazing wife Courtney, I love you beyond words and thank you so much for all of your support and for making me the luckiest guy in the world!

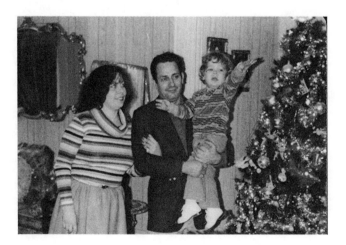

Contents

INTRODUCTION

PUTTING THE *HEART* BEFORE THE HORSE

"It's hard to beat a person who never gives up." —BABE RUTH

Everyone has a story to tell. I've poured out my heart and soul into this book to tell mine. I'm living proof that slow and steady *still* wins the race, that the American Dream is alive and well. You don't have to be the smartest or most talented person in the room to get ahead, just the one who wants it the most. No dream is too far-fetched, so long as you match it with sufficient grit, tenacity, unwavering focus, and plenty of thick skin. If I can do it, so can you!

My firsthand experience aside, it would seem that Babe Ruth was definitely onto something. His assertion sounds simple enough. Just keep at it, whatever "it" is, and sky's the limit! It's hard to argue with success, and, in Babe Ruth's case, this approach was so wildly successful that it transcended baseball and cemented his status among the most iconic sports heroes in American history. But if this strategy is so effective, why has unmet potential become so widespread? When did mediocrity become the status quo? What's holding so many of us back from chasing our dreams or living up to our full potential?

These troubling trends force us to reexamine my original premise. Maybe being "hard to beat" is not so simple after all. Perhaps my deductive reasoning was flawed, because I made the mistaken assumption that Babe Ruth's methodology was easily reproducible. Of course, it worked for Babe Ruth—he was *Babe Ruth!* According to this school of thought, Babe Ruth was no ordinary person. He was gifted with special physical talents; therefore, we can't use him as a point of reference. Like some comic book superhero or mythological god, his is an impossible standard to live up to…

So wait; not giving up also worked for me. Does that mean I'm special, too? Of course not, but that's the problem with this narrow-minded perspective. No one is inherently special, but we're all capable of greatness if we're willing to exert the necessary effort. It's self-serving to ascribe superhuman attributes to anyone that achieves extraordinary feats, because it gets you off the hook. Why bother swinging for the fences if you've already convinced yourself you don't have what it takes to be successful? You can't fail if you don't try at all, so you safely cling to the sidelines, watching others stick their necks out.

This is the crux of the problem. We are meant for more than passively floating through life. We've become too pragmatic and risk averse about our hopes and dreams. It's emblematic of modern society. This book will hopefully serve as a wake-up call and a call to arms to abandon passivity and to actively reclaim a victorious life!

The more things change, the more they remain the same.

On the one hand, we've all benefited tremendously from the tech boom. The ease and the convenience of the virtual reality we've grown accustomed to makes it seem like everything is just one "click" away. We want what we want, and we're entitled to getting it now, not tomorrow, and definitely not next week! And our fixation with prompt service extends well beyond the food and entertainment industry. By and large, we're beholden to the allure of overnight success, the quick fix, the life hack, and all manner of instant gratification. Why bother "paying your dues" or "fighting the good fight" when you can live the good life on easy street? Smooth sailing is the name of the game.

These are all signs of the times, but, thankfully, there's a lot that has indeed remained the same. Little kids' faces still light up when you ask them, "So what do you want to be when you grow up?" They're always ecstatic to share their amazingly cool dream of becoming—wait for it—an "ASTRONAUT!" The rousing announcement is typically met with heaps of boisterous praise and positive reinforcement. You're also bound to hear a, "You can do anything you set your mind to, buddy!" thrown in by one of the doting parents. The kid, of course, is still beaming and utterly convinced he's a lock for a future in space exploration. It's all very adorable, and I get a kick out of it every time.

Think back to the time when you were a child and you were asked that same timeless question. I'm willing to bet you also had big dreams. We all did! Nothing was out of bounds. Everything and anything was fair game. President, veterinarian, ballerina, you name it! So what happened? Our grandiose plans came crashing down to Earth. In their place, more-pedestrian, low-risk, low-reward pursuits. Living without a greater purpose, we fill this void with nonsense. But chances are that if you're like most people, there's that inner voice calling you to something greater, of substance.

Somewhere along the way, we tragically allowed our hopes and dreams to get stifled by the oppressive pragmatism we call reality, or adulthood. Or maybe we let others dictate what that reality was supposed to look like. We're flooded with glamourized examples of get-rich-quick schemes and instant celebrity. We're also fixated on certainty and avoiding the shame of failure. In the hustle and bustle of this fast-paced existence, you'd be crazy to waste years of your life chasing something, unless you were pretty certain that it was a sure bet in the long run or that your skills and talents aligned well with that endeavor. Doing so would be irrationally putting the proverbial cart before the horse or biting off more than you can chew.

Not to rain on anyone's parade, but I couldn't disagree more with that worldview. We owe it to ourselves to bring our "A" game, day in, day out. While there's no question that technology has come a long way, there's still no such thing as "success-on-demand." When it comes to achieving greatness or to making a genuine difference in the world, there are no shortcuts, fast tracks, or E-Z Passes. Now, more than ever, the adage of never giving up on your dreams holds all the more true. Many of us fail to launch our dreams because we've been brainwashed into accepting things as they are, settling for a life less lived, and barely scratching the surface of our ultimate capabilities.

Can you imagine telling that idealistic and impressionable younger you that the whole "astronaut thing" didn't work out so that, instead, you're in a dead-end, unfulfilling job, just counting the days until your retirement? The younger you starts crying hysterically—"Nice one, are you happy now?" Living a less than an ordinary life isn't anyone's destiny. To blaze your own trail, you're going to need to snap out of your trance and to assume direct oversight of your destiny. That idealistic little kid is still in there somewhere. The onus is on you to find him or her.

To that end, I opted to flip the script, putting my *heart* before the horse. No longer would I allow myself to be passively led by outside forces, like the passenger in a horse-drawn carriage. I assumed full control of my life, leading from the front, "the *Heart* Way." For the better part of the last thirty years, I kept at it, methodically plodding along the road less traveled, hoping against hope I could fulfill my dream. They said it couldn't be done. "A doctor? A heart surgeon? Come on, who are you kidding?" According to so-called conventional wisdom, I was ill-equipped to meet the challenge. My parents were "fresh off the boat," and our working-class, Cuban immigrant family could barely make ends meet. The socioeconomic chips were stacked against me, so I had to rely heavily on my heart for any shot at pulling off such an improbable upset!

But, much to the chagrin of countless naysayers and critics, I quietly persisted in actualizing my impossible dream, independently charting my own course, and grinding out the journey, one milestone at a time. This hard-fought rite of passage was an uphill climb through rugged terrain, in ceaselessly stormy weather. Rest stops were few and far between. To become a heart-transplant surgeon, I would have to successfully navigate the longest period of training required in any area of medicine. Only a chosen few are selected to endure this grueling decade of surgical residency beyond medical school. When it was all said and done, I finally made it to the finish line, and what started as an impossible dream became an ultimate reality!

This book, my story, begins and ends with the heart—the figurative or metaphysical heart. Where there's heart, there's a way. Heart conquers all. It's not a quantifiable trait. It won't show up on any stats sheet or any prefight "tale of the tape." But it's the reason why the odds-on favorite doesn't always win and why there's invariably a "Cinderella team" in every major athletic tournament. The reality is that, much like meteorologists, expert oddsmakers are never 100 percent accurate. All bets are off when you factor heart into your prediction model. That's why a "Cinderella team" still plays the games: no matter how lopsided the talent appears on paper or how heavily favored one combatant is relative to the other, it's the team with the most heart that may ultimately win the contest.

Take it from me: defying the odds and fulfilling your dreams comes down to going all in and never settling for anything less than your best effort. I call this living *"the Heart Way."* Be forewarned: this path is far from smooth sailing. There will be dark days, failures, and disappointments along the way. That's simply the nature of the beast, because the full scope of your inner greatness cannot be unleashed without your being pushed well beyond your comfort zone. Fair-weather dreamers abound. They talk a big game, daydreaming about being "x" or doing "y." But only a select few actually walk the walk and follow through with their plans. When the going gets tough, they don't throw in the towel, and their efforts never falter. You could say they're effectively *heart* to beat!

That's what my story is all about. To be clear, it's not just another book about medicine or surgery. If that were the case, I would have entitled it *Dazzling Digits,* as a satirical nod to Dr. Ben Carson's classic *Gifted Hands.* No, this is a book about heart, all heart everything, not heart surgery. The latter is simply the illustrative backdrop to chronicle my underdog story. As such, this book is really intended for all walks of life, to inject passion into the lives of those in desperate need of a driving force, to reinvigorate those who have lost it, or to embolden those who've been hesitant to go "all in." Maybe it can provide that key spark for those early in their quest or for those in a rut who need to reinvent themselves and to start anew. You can think of it as an inspirational guide, an anecdotal blueprint on how to meet the challenges or obstacles you encounter on your journey head-on and on how to cope with and to overcome the inevitable failures and hardships along the way, all the while maintaining your sanity and sense of humanity.

You see, I may be a heart surgeon by trade, but my story goes well beyond my professional identity. To reach this point in my life, I persevered through countless challenges while growing up in a Cuban immigrant family. Having defied the odds every step of the way, my life story is a testament to the American Dream, that success is not bestowed but earned by those with the greatest work ethic and the biggest heart. Throughout this book, I share the many life lessons learned along the way to help others push beyond their perceived limitations and reach their full potentials.

I don't pretend to have all the answers, nor do I profess to be an expert in the genre of self-help. When it comes to success and overcoming adversity, I can only share what did and didn't work for me. It's certainly not intended to be a one-size-fits-all account, generalizable to one and all. To flesh out the discussion and to provide a more comprehensive representation of the subject matter, I've sprinkled in the perspectives from quite a few experts and thought leaders spanning the fields of education, psychology, and sports. That should, hopefully, go a long way towards convincing you that not everything I've written in this book can be easily dismissed as the delusional ramblings of some arrogant surgeon.

Kidding aside, I promise to have your best interests at heart! As an added bonus, the final section of the book covers the essentials for maintaining a healthy heart and for maximizing your life expectancy. It's been said that the pen is mightier than the sword. In a similar vein, I hope the pen is likewise more impactful than the scalpel, yielding a more far-reaching benefit to the greatest number of people. Happy reading!

PART ONE

A *HEART* KNOCK LIFE: THE EARLY LESSONS

*"Working hard may help you maintain
To learn to overcome the heartaches and pain."*
–Wu-Tang Clan in "C.R.E.A.M."

"If you're not in it to win it, there's always plenty of room at the kids' table."

–BRIAN LIMA

CHAPTER 1

"THE HEART WAY" TO VICTORY

"What is stronger than the human heart which shatters over and over and still lives?" —Rupi Kaur

We've all been there—whether at home, growing up, or in grade school, getting scolded for bad behavior and being accused of preferring to learn things "the hard way." The "hard way," in this context, of course, refers to learning through trial and error and unpleasant experiences seared into our memories, like the one time I decided to pick up a stray cat by its tail so I could pet it. It seemed like an awesome idea at the time. I was seven years old, and, despite my mother's repeated warnings, I boldly embarked on this ill-fated mission, only to be met by all the vicious fury this ferocious little feline could muster. Innumerable leg lacerations and claw marks later, I learned the hard way that any attempt at tugging on a kitty's tail is dangerous business and should be avoided altogether.

As Shakespeare famously wrote in *The Tempest*, "The past

is prologue." Avoiding the mistakes of the past is a vital adaptation for future advancement. I guess that, in a perfect world, all of the amassed life lessons would be neatly catalogued and readily accessible so we could consciously avoid the hard way and live happily ever after. Not to be a Debbie Downer, but the reality is that we live in an imperfect world, full of well-meaning people but also plagued with egos, biases, corruption, and social injustices. To navigate and thrive in this hostile environment, there's no getting around having to get your hands dirty. After all, "you can't climb up the ladder of success with your hands in your pocket." (Arnold Schwarzenegger)

So, like it or not, life is a contact sport, and you really have to be all in it to win it. If you're not in it to win it, there's always plenty of room at the kids' table. This realization begs the question: how do we prepare for or cope with the inevitable failures and disappointments that come along the way? I've pondered this nagging question so many times throughout the years, frustrated by the lack of solutions the world had to offer. Until recently, my best answer(s) could be summed up with a colorful flurry of sports analogies and inspirational quotes, such as those from the iconic figures that I've included throughout this book. Take for instance, the elite NFL quarterback Tom Brady, arguably the best the game has ever seen. Having honed his capacity for selective amnesia, he can effortlessly forget he threw those four interceptions in the first half. By not dwelling on these flagrant mistakes, he can move forward, stay laser-focused, and still pull out the win for his team. Likewise, the world-class boxer in a championship bout has that "refuse-to-lose" mentality. He may get beaten or knocked out, but he'll go out swinging, never giving up, and protecting himself at all times (or trying to, at least).

While these are certainly worthwhile strategies and individuals to emulate, we may not necessarily have to look outward for sources of inspiration. What if I told you that the superhero alter ego you've been yearning to invoke has been right under your nose this whole time? I was struck by this epiphany during one of the heart-transplant procedures I performed last year. Immediately after I removed the recipient's old heart, it spontaneously continued to beat a few more times, as I held it in my hands, as if it wasn't quite ready to relinquish its important job just yet. Coincidentally, this also happened to be the very first heart transplant ever performed on Long Island, a huge milestone for the region and the proudest moment of my surgical career! So, given this momentous occasion, the procedure was being filmed, and, thankfully, this magical moment was captured on video to be shared with the world! (For access to the actual video footage, please visit https://youtu.be/HqY7NWorrpI) Not to be outdone, after I feverishly sewed in the new heart, it instinctively began beating right away, hours after being removed from the donor and transported to our hospital!

Just wow! It gets me every time, and it's why I do what I do. But something finally dawned on me, after so many years of soul searching, introspection, and chasing my dreams. It turns out that the ultimate, most relentless, inspirational force lies within us, beating in our chest, sustaining our very life—our heart! The veritable Energizer® bunny that is the human heart has Herculean physiologic prowess unmatched by any professional athlete or by any mere mortal, for that matter. You couldn't possibly ask for a better "ride-or-die" companion! Whether you're awake or asleep, happy or sad, nervous or afraid, your heart just keeps chugging along, beating about

100,000 times every day and roughly 2.5 billion times during your lifetime! Every minute, this little fist-sized muscle pumps 1.5 gallons of blood through a mind-boggling 60,000 miles of blood vessels. And, during pregnancy, the heart ups the ante even further, by doubling its pumping capability, to ensure that the developing fetus is getting enough blood flow.

Truth be told, as someone who's devoted much of my adult life to mastering the art of cardiac surgery and to taking care of the sickest of the sick heart patients, I'm clearly partial to the mystical wonder of the human heart. But, that aside, can you really blame me? I mean, seriously, no offense to my colleagues in other medical specialties, but when's the last time you heard anyone say, "I love you with all of my kidneys"?! Throughout human history, the heart has unquestionably garnered the most attention, as the most romanticized, idolized, and inspirational part of our body. Needless to say, the heart has all of the other organs *beat* (see what I did there?) by a mile. The allure of the heart simply cannot be denied.

But allow me to take it a step further. What if we approached life's challenges and setbacks just as our own hearts continuously strive to meet the demands of our bodies—unrelenting and with constant effort and action, even in dire circumstances? Rather than shying away from these obstacles or dwelling on our mistakes and misfortunes, what if we just kept methodically moving forward, onwards and upwards, without skipping a beat, focusing on what lies ahead and hellbent on conquering what we set out to accomplish? We could affectionately refer to this strategy as *"the Heart Way."*

The symbolic significance here cannot be overstated. By substituting the word "heart" for the word "hard," we are consciously nullifying the negative connotations of any challenging or unpleasant task. In so doing, we are effectively empowering ourselves to overcome that self-sabotaging force of inertia holding us hostage and preventing us from taking the pivotal first step towards fulfilling our dreams. Substituting the word "heart" also invigorates us to persist along this quest, when the going gets tough and we're tempted to throw in the towel. Pulling this off is admittedly much easier said than done, especially these days, where instant gratification has become everyone's top priority and entitlement. Virtually every want and need imaginable, from food to entertainment, is just one click away. To make matters worse, glamourized stories of overnight success, celebrity, and material wealth are endlessly streamed via social media. These household names have absurdly emerged as the new role models for our youth, prompting widespread repudiation of any course of action they deem even remotely difficult or unpleasant.

But make no mistake: a number of facts still hold true, no matter how topsy-turvy the world has become. Shortsighted, get-rich-quick schemes and other vapid pursuits, driven solely by selfish desires for fame and fortune, are ultimately unfulfilling. It's just how we're wired,—not to mention that prisons are full of convicts that opted for life in the fast lane. Our choices have consequences, and anything truly worth doing is not going to be easy. If it were easy, then everyone would do it. That's what makes the journey special and genuinely rewarding, so there's no use overthinking it any further. There are no shortcuts, easy ways out, or free lunches. I've come to find that *the Heart Way* is the only way.

"Nothing in the world is worth having or worth doing unless it means effort, pain, difficulty… I have never in my life envied a human being who led an easy life. I have envied a great many people who led difficult lives and led them well." –Theodore Roosevelt

To clarify, I'm not suggesting we all become masochistic gluttons for punishment. And neither was Theodore Roosevelt. Quite the contrary—life is about balance and moderation. There's a time and a place for leisure, letting your guard down, celebrating small victories, and enjoying precious moments with friends and family. Likewise, there's also a time to buckle down, to stare down your goals, and to launch headlong into battle with your obstacles, enduring all the gut-wrenching setbacks and failures along the way. By all intents and purposes, it seems the pendulum has swung disproportionately towards la-la land, following our increasingly hedonistic tendencies. This principle of balance holds universally true for both our physical and metaphorical hearts. Take, for instance, our diet. As much as I'd love to sugarcoat it, a heart-healthy diet doesn't quite hit the spot like a nice juicy steak or a heaping bowl of pasta. Every now and again, sure! I'll allow myself the indulgence. Call it a "cheat day," a "cheat meal," or, more generically, "delayed gratification." But we all know that, just as with smoking cigarettes, eating this way on a regular basis would be quite hazardous to our health.

As the diet example illustrates, there are countless, painful choices we must make for our greater good, be it for our overall health or to further our quest for success. These daily choices often entail delayed gratification, gritty determination, and willpower to forego the path of least resistance and all of its shiny distractions and temptations. For the better part of my late teens, twenties, and thirties, I sacrificed tirelessly to stay on course. I kept my eyes on the prize. When my counterparts were out partying, clubbing, or sleeping in, I was chipping away at my dream, one assignment at a time, class after class, semester after semester, year after year. Had I not invested this time and effort, I can assure you I would have never become the heart surgeon, or that man, that I am today.

When you deviate from *the Heart Way*, the repercussions can be catastrophic, even fatal, in all phases of your life. Your heart's only job is to keep beating, to keep you alive, moment after moment, until you take your final, dying breath. But not all hearts have the same physiologic capacity or level of efficiency. Like us, they aren't invincible. They're vulnerable to the cumulative effects of our unhealthy practices and dietary choices. Unable to circulate adequate blood supply, a damaged heart may not be able to meet the demands of our body. This is a precarious predicament to be in—hence, the phrase, "as serious as a heart attack." It may unfold gradually, with plaque buildup causing progressive narrowing of the heart arteries over time. Conversely, it may occur suddenly, if a "widow-maker" blood clot abruptly shuts down a major blood vessel in the heart. Whatever the case may be, these disastrous events are largely avoidable, if we strictly adhere to preventative measures and optimal lifestyle modifications proven to be effective.

My father suffered a life-threatening heart attack in his early fifties, when I was only ten years old. At that point in my young life, it was the biggest scare I or anyone in our family had ever experienced. We were terrified and felt utterly helpless. He was the center of our universe, and life without him was unfathomable. The years of fatty foods and high-salt intake prominently featured in our Cuban cuisine had caught up with him. As a perfect case study in what not to do, our family's version of "primary care" was getting rushed to the emergency room only when we were violently ill. For many Latino families and other members of the community sharing our lower socioeconomic demographic, this is, unfortunately, standard operating procedure. Annual checkups and cancer screening? No thanks. It begs the question: Maybe if my mother had undergone her screening colonoscopy when she was fifty, she wouldn't have died of metastatic colon cancer at the age of sixty-five? Maybe she would have seen me finish my decade-long surgical training and finally let me take care of her for a change? I guess we'll never know, but these lingering questions will undoubtedly torment me the rest of my days…

Luckily, my father was successfully treated with a noninvasive balloon angioplasty procedure. He didn't get off so easy the next time, when a sextuple bypass (that's not a typo—six bypasses) open heart operation was required to reestablish adequate blood flow, to save his ailing heart fifteen years later. He lived another twelve years, but he was never really the same. This traumatic experience left an indelible mark on me, impacting not only my career trajectory but also how I approach my own health. My family didn't know any better, but I do! The least I can do is to make leading a healthy lifestyle a major priority in my life, and I have. And for my patients, or for anyone who will listen (you included), I further honor my parents' memory by promoting best practices for healthy living.

The moral of the story is that a healthy heart will not falter. It will not hesitate or agonize over whether or not to beat. It just beats, no matter the circumstances. Think of how more productive and resilient we would be or how much simpler life itself would become, if we just reflexively acted more and hesitated less. In the face of stress, hardship, tragedy, or failure, we would just proactively keep on trucking, instead of waving the white flag. Less time would be wasted wallowing in self-pity or perseverating over our mistakes, the opinions of others, or how we will be perceived. There's no telling how far we could reach or how little would be beyond our grasp. Like the powerful heart of an elite athlete, forged by deliberate exposure to grueling levels of physical stress, our metaphorical hearts could be engineered to withstand the worst life could throw our way yet still claim victory. As we plod along, battle after battle, our endurance builds, and our confidence, resilience, and grit accumulate. Trying circumstances become effortlessly manageable, formidable tasks seemingly surmountable. Success becomes habitual. This is living *the Heart Way*.

Obviously, this doesn't happen overnight. It takes time. No one is born with the heart of a world-class cyclist or marathon runner. No one is born a master chess player, a concert pianist, or a Superbowl MVP. I wasn't born being able to do heart surgery. What's the common denominator? It's a process. You must be willing to relentlessly and repeatedly push yourself well beyond your comfort zone and skill set. It's all about the reps, the "10,000-hour rule," as we'll get into. That's the story of my life, and that's what this book is all about. That's how I became heart to beat! In the chapters that follow, I will share how this all unfolded in somewhat chronological order. I will share key takeaways from my biggest victories and defeats, my saddest and happiest moments, and the how, the what, and the why of *the Heart Way*.

For now, I'll leave you with this handy mnemonic that summarizes the salient features of *the Heart Way*. Think of it as a constellation of overlapping themes and attributes that syner-gistically produce a blueprint for success. I'll periodically refer back to it, as we cover relevant topics.

The H.E.A.R.T. Way:

H: Hard Work—the foundation of all success

E: Eager—being positively energetic; smiling in the face of misery, being optimistic and ambitious; having a growth mindset; being entrepreneurial

A: Aligned—being in sync with your purpose, with the big picture, and with your moral compass; having gravitas, being *anchored*, being grounded; never settling, having no complacency; always taking the high road

R: Resolute—being purposeful and unrelenting; being gritty; being disciplined; being committed to getting better (self-improvement)

T: Thoughtfulness—as in mindfulness; self-awareness; emotional intelligence; being in the moment, thinking of the good things for which to be thankful; thinking of other's feelings and needs, being empathetic

"To elevate your game, you must eliminate your doubt."

–BRIAN LIMA

CHAPTER 2

HEART OVER MATTER: YOU ARE THE MASTER

"I am not what has happened to me. I am what I choose to become." –CARL JUNG

"You must expect great things of yourself before you can do them." –MICHAEL JORDAN

One of my favorite movies while growing up was Berry Gordon's *The Last Dragon,* a cult classic featuring Leroy Green (aka "Bruce Leeroy"), a young martial artist desperately seeking his idol Bruce Lee's level of mastery. A true master, Leroy's teacher explains, exudes a visible, mystical "glow" over his entire body. Leroy sets out on a spiritual quest to unlock this special power. During the movie's climactic finale, Leroy has to do battle with his arch nemesis, the villainous gang leader, Sho'nuff. Things aren't going well for Leroy, who's on the receiving end of a vicious beating by Sho'nuff, who demands that Leroy acknowledge him as the true master. At that very moment, Leroy's life flashes before his eyes, and he finally realizes that, all along, he had already achieved master status. He just didn't know it, until now. When Sho'nuff asks him for the last time, "WHO'S THE MASTER?!" Leroy defiantly declares, "I AM!" Then he instantly shows off his newfound glow and defeats Sho'nuff. The rest is movie history.

While I still haven't been able to convince my wife to watch this cinematic classic, I'm holding out hope she'll eventually have a change of heart and *see the light*. Notwithstanding, there's a lot to unpack and learn from Leroy's quest for mastery. Many of us have allowed our own insecurities, past experiences, skewed view of the world, or outright fear to limit our growth and potential, and we continue to do so. We just haplessly stay in our lane, sticking to what's familiar and comfortable. This self-sabotage is often further compounded by the lame advice and sentiments peddled by our friends, our family, and our coworkers. They reaffirm our preconceived notions or tell us precisely what we want to hear. No surprise there. Chances are their brains are hopelessly mired in the same tangled mess that's weighing us down. By selling ourselves short, we end up settling for a life less lived, accepting the fate of unmet potential, and taking up permanent residence in the land of status quo. Lackadaisical effort leads to lackluster results and lukewarm reception, a vicious cycle set on autoloop. This self-fulfilling prophecy comes to define our life.

Does it really need to be this way? Not at all. So how do we break the cycle? What's holding you back from fulfilling your dream(s), from getting that promotion, or from getting that dream job? As you might have guessed by now, the answer is relatively simple. It starts with you! You are the master! You are the key to your success and the only way out of your personal jam. The biggest threat to your success is staring at you in the mirror. You have to get out of your head, get into the game, and take ownership of your life's direction. "The answer," as author Gary John Bishop bluntly states, is, "not out there, but inside yourself. It's not that you have to find the answer, you are the answer...people spend their lives waiting for the cavalry, all the while never realizing they are the cavalry. Your life is waiting on you to finally show up."

The rate-limiting step in accomplishing your goal(s) or in unleashing your full potential is owning that you, and you alone, are responsible for how much or how little you achieve in this life. My life story is a testament to the power of this critical realization. No one, myself included, would have ever predicted that a kid from a working-class, Cuban immigrant family could get educated and trained at some of the most prestigious universities in the world, becoming a leading cardiac surgeon in the fields of heart failure and heart transplant. In fact, if you had approached me during my teenage years in New Jersey, alerting me of this eventuality, I would have likely retorted, "Get outta hea!!! What are you? Some kinda comedian or something?! Fogettaboutit!"—in a very thick Jersey accent.

This brings me to the beginning of my personal journey I would like to share with you. My parents and two older siblings (Edward and Diana) were forced to flee their home in Cuba because of Fidel Castro's oppressive Communist regime. Once Castro took power in 1959, his government seized the Lima family farm, "La Fortuna," and later imprisoned two of my dad's brothers for their political views. In a desperate attempt to save his family from these deplorable conditions, my father courageously moved the Lima clan to America in 1968, onboard one of the Freedom Flights. They were among the estimated 300,000 refugees that fled Cuba, seeking political asylum, the largest airborne refugee operation in U.S. history. Broke and unable to speak a lick of English, my college-educated father had to secure any job he could it get. It was a demanding and unpleasant job in Newark, New Jersey, at a pigment factory, where he worked countless overtime shifts to put food on the table.

By the time I came along in 1976, my siblings were already teenagers, and the family had settled in the town of Kearny, New Jersey, a suburb of Newark with a clear view of the Manhattan skyline. Kearny is a blue-collar, working-class town, whose most recent claim to fame was being a main location for the filming of the hit HBO series, *The Sopranos*. We lived in a small, three-bedroom apartment on the ground floor of a three-story building.

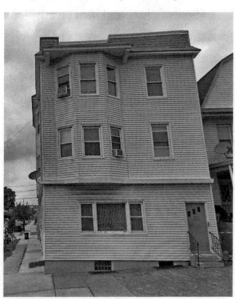

My apartment (first floor), while I was growing up in Kearny, New Jersey.

Edward and Diana each had their own room, which unfortunately meant I had to sleep on a bed in my parent's bedroom until my sophomore year of high school, when Diana moved in with her fiancé. We spoke only Spanish at home, and, apart from what I had picked up while watching cartoons, I didn't formally learn English until kindergarten. The importance of both education and our Catholic faith prompted my parents to initially send me to St. Cecilia's, a local parochial school. My earliest recollections of St. Cecilia's were far from that of a model student. I was repeatedly chastised by my teachers for not paying attention, for being fidgety or having "ants in my pants," for not following directions, and for other behavioral indicators of a child with attention deficit hyperactivity disorder (ADHD). Back then, however, prescribing medications like Ritalin was not yet a widely accepted treatment option. My parents were none the wiser.

My mother barely had a high school education, but she was an amazing homemaker and a doting mom. To help make ends meet, she would do some babysitting, and, along with my dad, she would help a local food vendor by painstakingly chopping up slabs of beef and putting them on sticks to make shish kebabs, for hours on end. My parents went above and beyond to provide for us, leaving no stone unturned or unclaimed overtime shifts on the table. In spite of these colossal efforts, however, they, sadly, could no longer afford the nominal tuition at St. Cecilia's. After fifth grade, I had to transfer to a nearby public school to finish out sixth through eighth grades. In retrospect, this turned out to be a somewhat traumatic transition for me. Leaving behind the comfort and familiarity of St. Cecilia's, along with my close group of friends, was a scary proposition.

Slight tangent: Did I mention how ridiculously delectable my mother's home-cooked Cuban food was? Let's just say that I never skipped a meal and that the portion size was equivalent to the maximum quantity of food that could be forcibly heaped on my plate. Suffice it to say that I had managed to pack on enough pounds to catapult me into the "husky" size category for kid's clothing. Having to transfer schools and start all over as the chubby new kid was no cakewalk.

For starters, I ended up getting dragged into a bunch of fights in sixth grade, not by choice but purely out of self-defense. Any real bully worth his weight in salt has to test the moxie of the new kid, and I was the main course for this juvenile rite of passage. Kids can be difficult, and if you've ever experienced bullying, you know what I mean. But it is those experiences that can make you stronger or that, perhaps, can give you the resilience and the determination to prove the bullies wrong about your moxie.

It turns out that all that baby fat I was lugging around came in handy. In what can only be described as some rudimentary form of Sumo wrestling, I managed to rack up a respectable winning record, by leveraging my disproportionate weight advantage. This strategy served me well, until one seasoned combatant pinpointed the glaring weakness in my defensive stance. He connected squarely on my nose with a viciously telegraphed haymaker, and it bled profusely. The sight of my own blood sent me into a panic, and I began crying hysterically. This clearly did not help my bid for street cred.

The taunts and the bullying persisted, and my parents' broken English was also not spared from ridicule. To make matters worse, I was not very athletic and was always picked last for games. Unlike a lot of the other younger kids in the neighborhood, I was never involved in any organized sports, like Little League Baseball, Pop Warner football, or CYO (Catholic Youth Organization) basketball. For my parents, this simply wasn't a priority, not even a blip on their radar, and justifiably so…They had a lot on their plate already. It was around this time when my brother Ed began having his psychotic breaks, culminating in a diagnosis of paranoid schizophrenia. He was in graduate school, studying for his master's in teaching, when things came to a head.

My brother's battle with schizophrenia is something I rarely share with others. In fact, I debated long and hard about whether or not to include it in this book. I love my brother, and, to this day, I continue supporting him and doing whatever I can to ensure his safety and well-being. In the end, I decided that his story needed to be told because of its fundamentally critical and overarching relevance to my story, my upbringing, and my family's saga of hardship and sacrifice. Omitting it would be a weak move, reverting back to my timid former self, nervously evasive or immaturely overcome with shame and resentment whenever my friends would ask, "What's up with your brother? He's kind of weird." Leaving out his story would be disingenuous, a true injustice to the struggles he's had and continues to endure. It would feed into the lingering taboo that is mental illness, further marginalizing those afflicted. As I witnessed firsthand, this holds especially true in my Latino culture, where mental illness continues to be vilified and to be judged within a context of religious undertones.

Before and periodically after my brother was "formally" diagnosed with schizophrenia, my family was convinced that satanic possession was the likely culprit for his debilitating sickness. A number of "exorcisms" and spiritual interventions were attempted. but to no avail. These shenanigans did, however, successfully scare the living daylights out of me, as it would have scared any kid my age. Just as with my father's heart attack, we were helpless. We didn't know any better. Ed lived at home with us, but, for the most part, he confined himself to his room, preferring solitude over the company of others. On a few occasions, he would drag his mattress into my parents' bedroom at night, because he was terrified of all the voices he was hearing and all the hallucinations he couldn't shake.

Not fully grasping the severity of his illness, we kept hoping Ed would just miraculously snap out of it, my dad especially. In good faith, he made numerous attempts at nudging Ed into some semblance of adulthood. There was the job at the supermarket, working at the cash register, and a job at my dad's factory, working as a laboratory technician. Ed would last for a couple of days, but, invariably, he was no match for the mounting storm of stress and anxiety wreaking havoc on his mind. Time and time again, he would just abruptly leave, triggering a frantic phone call to the house, alerting us of yet another devastating setback. My parents grew so desperate they sought out help from a Santero, an Afro-Cuban witch doctor of sorts, who recommended they take some of Ed's clothes and belongings, wrap them up, and toss them in the Passaic River. They did just that, were seen by police, and were nearly arrested!

Meanwhile, despite all the turmoil, my parents somehow managed to always keep a good face on. Preserving the sanctity of our home and family was their top priority, and their track record was beyond reproach. Not once did they skimp on their parental duties, showering me with boundless love and affection. Their benevolence was a constant force that steadied me through these stormy times. I vividly recall my father telling me to work hard and to stay focused every chance he could get. He was a stern, yet loving, family man who could make you laugh but could make you listen, at the same time. He was intense, but in a good way! This gifted storyteller would regularly sit me down at the kitchen table for these deep talks—countless sessions of him giving me life lessons and the raw and unfiltered facts about human nature, preparing me for the harsh realities of our society. He told me that no one is more inherently special or more talented or more gifted or smarter than anyone else. No one is destined for greatness. He told me that the one who succeeds is the person who's willing to put in the time and the work to do so, and the person who wants success more than anyone else. A strong work ethic was the ultimate talent. He would implore me to seize the opportunities he never had so that I didn't end up like him, working under horrible conditions inhaling toxic fumes at a pigment factory. He gave me the courage and inspiration to think big, to swing for the fences, and to look beyond my immediate surroundings and circumstances.

He lit the fire in my belly.

This fire, however, lay dormant for a time, relegated to back burner status, as I coasted through middle school and junior high. Then came my eighth-grade graduation ceremony, a pivotal and defining moment of my life, when all of Dad's lessons hit me like a ton of bricks. Gerard, one of my closest friends and my eventual best man, earned a ton of awards—in math, in science, you name it—he won it. He was even called on stage several times, and as the teacher handing out the awards delivered accolades, I felt myself shrinking, sinking deeper and deeper into my seat. I totally blew it! I felt ashamed and utterly humiliated. How could I let this happen? He was from a family of immigrants, too. He wasn't wealthy, and he wasn't more advantaged than me, and the only thing he did better than me was work harder. This was a defining moment that impacted the rest of my life. The proverbial switch was flipped. This sobering revelation instantaneously and irrevocably transformed my worldview. I had not done my best, not even close to it, and that's never okay.

As I watched him accept those awards, my stoic exterior concealed my inconsolable guilt and the boulder in the pit of my stomach. This façade proved to be very effective, I must say. My parents never suspected anything was awry. All they had ever asked of me was to do my best. After everything they had done for me and after all the trials and tribulations they had suffered, my best was the very least I could do. Not unreasonable or overbearing in the slightest, they never specifically demanded straight As, nor were they at all disappointed with my mediocre showing that fateful night. Why this one event became such an impactful epiphany remains a mystery to me. But, for whatever the reason, one thing is for certain. It rekindled my dormant flame and awoke an *urgency of purpose* that thrust me forward, like a jet-fueled turbo boost. Without it, I might have never resolved to work so hard or commit myself to success. I never again wanted to feel that sting of defeat because I let laziness get the best of me. I didn't deserve to win anything that night. Gerard did, because he had his priorities straight and work ethic intact. It was time to go back to the drawing board, to retrace my missteps, and to orchestrate my triumphant comeback. Tapping into this newfound mind-set, I was going to hit the ground running in high school, determined to be the best. In the ensuing chapters, I'll share how that all came to fruition.

For now, let's recap the ground we've covered thus far. I think you'd agree that the socioeconomic chips were definitely stacked against me. Statistically speaking, I was a long shot, to say the least. That's the beauty of it. I'm living proof that the *American Dream* is not just some hokey catchphrase blurted out in political speeches. It's alive and well. That's all well and good, but you have to bear in mind that you're not entitled to the American Dream. It's a meritocracy, after all. To the victor belong the spoils, and victory is seldom, if ever, bestowed. It's earned, through blood, sweat, and tears, as my father painstakingly instilled in me at a very young age. My American Dream was not preordained, nor was I born an anointed prodigy or intellectual genius. No, I'm not special. I scratched and clawed my way to the top, every step of the way.

Here's a news flash: you're not special, either! Practically speaking, we are all the same. We are all subject to the same finicky, impatient, and hypercritical court of public opinion: "What have you done for me, lately?" But take solace in that while no one is special, everyone is capable. Yes, I know that, nowadays, we're supposed to believe we're all special. Suggesting otherwise would seem heretical or degrading to many. The PC police may be beating down my door, but don't shoot the messenger—I'm just calling it like I see it. If you want to find out just how "not special" you are, try cutting someone off on the freeway, stealing someone's parking spot at the mall, or dillydallying at a stoplight, as you scroll through your FB newsfeed! Yes, road rage is the ultimate reality check, a fascinating, yet unflinching, look into the truly harsh reality of our society. Even sweet ole Grannie will honk her horn and flip you the bird, if you pull one of these driving stunts.

These same primal instincts we all harbor are also readily apparent through the prism of professional sports. Last week, he scored the game-winning touchdown, so he's the toast of the town, "maybe the best ever," and "hall-of-fame bound," according to the commentators and sports columnists. This week, he fumbled the snap in the waning seconds, so the game was lost. Now we're all shouting expletives at the TV and clamoring for his dismissal; the home crowd is booing; the pundits are breaking down his flaws and wondering if the backup should take over next week. I think you get the picture. No matter who we are, we're only as good as our last mistake. The world could care less that we're just trying our best or that a singular event or poor performance could ever really define us. You don't get participation trophies in the real world. Swift and merciless "justice" awaits anyone who fails to deliver top quality, who wastes precious milliseconds of our time, or who just rubs us the wrong way.

I share these unpleasantries not to deter or to discourage you from chasing your dreams. My objective, instead, is to disclose the rules of engagement, the nature of the beast, if you will, so that you tread carefully on your path, aware and prepared for the inherent challenges that lie ahead. As Sun Tzu preaches in the *Art of War*, "If you know the enemy and know yourself, you need not fear the result of a hundred battles." Better yet, expect and prepare for the worst-case scenario. The best hitters in baseball know this all too well, anticipating that every pitcher they face is gunning to strike them out. No matter who you are, life will inevitably throw you curveballs or changeups, or it will bring you the heat with a one-hundred-mile-per-hour fastball. If you think you're special, stop kidding yourself. Don't fall into that trap. Am I special because

I'm a heart surgeon? No. Even when I conduct a technically perfect operation, the risk of death is ever present. If I lose a patient and have to break the terrible news to their family, do you really think they care if I "tried my best"? Of course not. Why should they?

We are the same. Or let's just say we all start out the same. We all start out with the possibility that you can be anything you want to be and that you can accomplish anything you want to accomplish. Along the way, all people make choices in their lives, and these choices will always have a big impact on their futures. Some choices inch you closer to your dreams, and some further away from them. Every day, I am reminded of this when I'm waiting, like everyone else in line, for my Venti Latte. No one knows you're a heart surgeon or a CEO or anything else special. You're just another person in line, who gets dirty looks if it takes you more than two seconds to order your expresso. This is a wake-up call for me every day—we are all the same. We are all the masters of our own destinies and the keys to our individual successes. Take a minute. Let those words sink in, and don't fret—you've got this!

"Visualize.
Actualize.
Repeat."
–BRIAN LIMA

CHAPTER 3

*HEART*IFICIAL INTELLIGENCE: POOR MAN'S GENIUS

*"We like to think of our champions and idols as superheroes, who were born different from us. We don't like to think of them as relatively ordinary people who made themselves extraordinary." –*CAROL S. DWECK

*"For me, the starting point for everything—before strategy, tactics, theories, managing, organizing, philosophy, methodology, talent, or experience—is work ethic. Without one of significant magnitude you're dead in the water, finished."–*BILL WALSH

When I meet people for the first time and when they learn of my background and journey, they often remark, "Wow! You must be really smart!" Flattered by the complimentary assumption, I politely smile and reply, "Thank you, but not exactly! I just worked really hard." The ensuing moments of awkward silence are always a dead giveaway that my sincere and self-deprecating response was not at all what they had expected to hear. You see, there's this prevailing misconception out there about successful people. For whatever reason, the cosmos has handpicked these special individuals—lucky winners of a genetic lottery, endowing them with superhuman attributes and talents. There's no use even trying if you don't already have "it." You'll never get there, no matter how hard you try. So stick with the peanut gallery, where you can play it safe, and critique the ones who dare enter the fray. Well, if that's how you see things, then I'm really sorry. You've missed the boat, because nothing can be further from the truth.

The truth is I've just never really viewed myself as "smart" per se. Don't get me wrong: I have an above-average IQ, but it's definitely not off the charts or genius level, by any stretch of the imagination. I also don't have a photographic memory, a bummer, for sure, as it would have come in really handy during college and medical school. And when it came to standardized tests, I could crack high enough scores after intense preparation, but never to the point of acing them with near-perfect marks. Purely and simply, I just outworked my peers at every level. Whether it was high school, college, or beyond, there were always students that were a good deal smarter than me: with a higher IQ or with highly coveted photographic memories. To compensate for my deficits, I had to rely on brute force and inspired performance. Inordinate amounts of time and effort were expended to cram facts and figures into my thick skull, and real estate was at a premium in this limited space.

You could say my secret weapon was getting "high," not high, as in the consumption of a mind-altering substance, but "H.I."—as in *Heartificial Intelligence*. Not to be confused with John C. Havens recent book, *Heartificial Intelligence: Embracing Our Humanity to Maximize Machines,* the kind of H.I. I'm referring to has a completely different connotation. I've coined H.I., in this context, as a lighthearted reference to circumventing my lack of true brilliance. Not to mention, it conveniently has the word "heart" spliced into it, which, in case you haven't noticed by now, is a major theme of this book and my life. The basic premise behind this workaround is that you need only to be smart enough, counterbalancing the rest with hard work, by essentially putting the "H" in *the Heart Way.* In his thought-provoking book, *Outliers,* Malcolm Gladwell expounds further on this notion, explaining that "a basketball player only has to be tall enough—and the same is true of intelligence. Intelligence has a threshold…Success is a function of persistence and doggedness and the willingness to work hard for twenty-two minutes to make sense of something that most people would give up on after thirty seconds."

Are you willing the put in the extra time and effort to learn and master a subject or a discipline, even if takes you much longer than your peers? Wait, let me guess. Some of you may be enamored with the motto, "work smarter, not harder," and feel utterly perplexed by my silly question. Quite frankly, I cringe whenever I hear that phrase, whose original meaning, I believe, has been grossly distorted into thinly veiled revelations of indolence and mischief. In my experience, it's become synonymous with shirking responsibility. Please disregard my cynicism, as it leaps off this page, but it totally sounds like something Ferris Bueller would have said during his epic day off, playing hooky, while smirking at the camera. So this is why I like to describe people who throw around this phrase as "too cool for school." They typically use it to punctuate their "I only need a C on the final to pass the class" dissertations we've all been subjected to, their delusional ramblings on the bare minimum required to eke by. Maybe it's also what all those students and parents were touting in that recent college scandal, falsifying applications and hiring mercenary test takers to ace the SAT (ouch, too soon?). You can see how well "working smarter" worked out for them. I'm not knocking efficiency or strategic time management, but don't be fooled—being smart and working hard are never mutually exclusive.

Back to my original question: are you willing to put in the work? I was. Fresh off the heels of the fiasco that was my eighth-grade graduation, I entered Kearny High School (KHS), no-holds-barred and with a chip on my shoulder. It was time to walk the walk and to see what I was capable of pulling off. This time, I would not be denied. I was going to hit the books hard, with a ferocity unmatched by any of my three hundred plus classmates, including my buddy, Gerard. In a way, I have him to thank for inspiring me to bring my "A" game to KHS. Every night, and with machinelike precision, I would voraciously devour my homework assignments and pore over my study notes for up to six hours. On exam days, I'd allot additional time in the early morning hours before school, a final walk through before the big game. My mother, God bless her soul, was my fail-safe alarm clock. No matter how early I "set the alarm," she'd lovingly wake me with a glass of hot chocolate and fresh toast! She was my biggest cheerleader.

Through trial and error, I gradually amassed an armamentarium of bare-knuckle study tactics, the most fine-tuned of which was rote memorization. The key, I discovered, was to methodically condense all of the relevant material to be tested on a "cheat sheet," using very tiny handwriting to fit as much information on as little paper as possible. This tedious exercise, in and of itself, would magically facilitate retention and regurgitation of the subject matter at test time. Psychologically speaking, there was the added benefit of whittling down a mountain of information into a more manageable synopsis. By rendering the task less daunting, I would feel confident about my chances for a successful outcome. After reading through my cheat sheet a few times, I was golden. It stuck in my head. Over time, I implemented my own shorthand for this homegrown microscribing to help streamline the process even further. And before long, I hit my stride, scoring at or near 100 percent on every test, and A+ in every class.

On one occasion, I walked into my freshman algebra classroom a few minutes early, as the teacher was erasing a problem on the chalkboard (remember those?) left over from an earlier calculus class. I remember staring at that incomprehensible alphabet soup in complete awe, wondering how on earth I would ever be able to tackle something of that complexity. It seemed so out of my league. Sensing my despair and impending panic attack, the seasoned teacher glanced over to me and allayed my fears. I can't recall precisely what she said, but, given her penchant for witty banter, it was something to the effect of, "Be patient, grasshopper. You'll get there soon enough." Sure, I had my doubts. But as I progressed through algebra, geometry, trigonometry, and finally calculus, her sage advice proved to be prophetic. Following this ordered succession of increasing complexity got me right to the place where I needed to be, just as it had for everyone else before me. The one exception, obviously, would be Isaac Newton, the guy who actually invented calculus to derive the laws of physics. But that's neither here nor there. You catch my drift. For us ordinary folk, the path to advanced levels of complexity and expertise, whether it be calculus or cardiac surgery, involves successive building blocks and growing pains. As Confucius says, "a journey of a thousand miles begins with a single step." Don't psyche yourself out or get intimidated before you even take your first step. Give yourself more credit. There's nothing special about the people that did it before you. Your Heartificial Intelligence will get you there, so just trust the process, and embrace the pain!

By now, you may be wondering if I actually had a life during high school. That's a legitimate question, with an answer that may surprise you. When I wasn't studying like a maniac, you would've probably found me in the high school weight room or on the football field. Let me explain. You see, apart from academics, I also decided to take aim at athletics with my entry into KHS, namely football. Football had become, far and away, my favorite sport. Whether it was two-hand touch or full-on tackle football, I had a blast playing with my buddies. We marveled at the incredible athleticism of the NFL elite. Star players, like Lawrence Taylor and Bo Jackson, seemed larger than life, modern day superheroes that clashed like arena gladiators every Sunday. To be good, of course, meant that you were big and strong, agile and fast—all the things I wasn't, yet.

If that all weren't motivation enough, I caught wind of some vicious rumors about the savage hazing that incoming fresh-men were subjected to, like getting stuffed into lockers and other unspeakable humiliations. My sister and older cousins were KHS alum and corroborated the veracity of these rumors. They shared firsthand accounts of their own horrific experiences. Seriously? I was not about to let anyone stuff me in a locker. Been there, done that, and I was over it! Historically, the perpetrators of these heinous acts were the bigger, stronger upperclassmen, most notably the football players. Say it ain't so! My imagination ran away with me. I kept having disturbing visions of "Ogre," from another 1980s movie gem, *Revenge of the Nerds,* screaming "NERRRRRRRRRRRDS!!!!!!" as I helplessly hung upside down in my locker. Hell, no! Enough was enough. Unlike the feeble geeks who waited until the end of the movie to stand up to the bullying jocks, I was going to meet the challenge head-on. Someway, somehow, I was going to will myself into jockhood, if it was the last thing I ever did. I vowed to erase the years of athletic ineptitude and ridicule that had plagued me in the past. My mission was to obliterate the dichotomy between nerd and jock and to turn the whole social order on its head.

Sound far-fetched? Maybe. The tale of the tape would have certainly argued that just my lettering in varsity football was a pipe dream, let alone the prospect of making any local headlines as a standout player. Our high school played in arguably the most competitive conference in the state of New Jersey, which included perennial powerhouse programs like those at Union and Elizabeth. I was a total newbie to the nitty gritty X's and O's, having never played a single down of organized football. Clocking in at five seconds flat in the forty-yard dash, I was also as slow as molasses. As I entered high school, a growth spurt had, fortunately, thinned out my pudgy frame. But, at six feet tall and weighing only 150 pounds, I was hardly a menacing force to be reckoned with on the football field. Lacking most of the physical and mental prerequisites for success at football, I faced an uphill battle to fulfill my quest.

My parents thought I was absolutely insane for wanting

to play this "barbaric" sport, but they humored me. I was allowed to play, but they never came to any games, refusing to be complicit in any of the injuries I would assuredly sustain. This endeavor was my pet project, and mine alone. During the summer leading up to my freshman year, I regularly worked out in the high school weight room, alongside many of the football players. It was intimidating and scary, but, surprisingly, I felt welcomed to this new home away from home. I took to powerlifting like a fish to water, adhering closely to the program the head coach had written up for the players. Slowly but surely, I was getting stronger. The coaches took notice, and I was among a handful of other "frosh" (incoming freshman) invited to attend summer training camp for the varsity football team. And so it began.

Leading up to the first day of class, this hellish two-week camp was the most physically grueling challenge I had ever faced. It's when I learned the true meaning of Vince Lombardi's oft-quoted phrase: "Fatigue makes cowards of us all." These three-a-day practice sessions spanned the entire day, from sunup to sundown, during the peak summer heat. We often were in "full pads" (helmet, shoulder pads, and the rest), dripping gallons of sweat, as we ran wind sprints and agility drills and hit tackling dummies, blocking sleds, or each other. It amazes me that none of us suffered serious heat exhaustion or dehydration, as we roasted under the scorching hot sun all those hours, wearing all that gear. To this day, I still can't stop thinking about those football camp days whenever I smell freshly cut grass.

Yes, on paper, it all sounds pretty awful. But, in actuality, this experience yielded a treasure trove of success habits I would carry with me for years to come. I could fill an entire book with the priceless life lessons I picked up during my stint in football jockdom. Together with his crew of henchmen—I mean, assistant coaches—our head coach doled out the virtues of tough love, discipline, teamwork, and accountability, to name a few, as a steady barrage with endless ammunition. Football training camp was the place where I learned that you can't take criticism personally, especially when engaging in full-on *heart-to-heart* combat. You must have thick skin. If you don't have it, then you better get some, ASAP! It's the only way you'll find out what's holding you back so you can inch closer to where you need to be. If you missed a blocking assignment, you got an earful from the coaches, in front of everyone, out in the open. All the players were held to account on their individual responsibilities and contributions both to the team and to every single play in the playbook. There was a zero-tolerance policy for laziness or tardiness. Any drill or play that was not executed to perfection would be repeated until it was flawless, no matter how many times were necessary to get it right. Repetition was the mission, perfection our obsession, and victory our only redemption.

Through football, you learned the critical difference between being hurt versus being injured. An actual injury means you are physically incapable of playing. If you're just "hurt," though, you can still play! You play through the pain and fatigue, for your team, for the win. You may get beaten, but you always refuse to lose. If you get tossed around like a rag doll or if your clock gets cleaned on a pummeling tackle, you get right back up. There's no crying or quitting in football, and the play doesn't end until the whistle blows. Football is a game of inches; therefore, attention to detail and minimizing mental mistakes are the keys to victory. The same applies to life. It's not about who is more talented. It's all about who can more consistently deliver perfect form and technique. Sure, you may think this all sounds like some macho mumbo jumbo. But's it not. Little did I know that many, if not all, of these indelible lessons would resurface throughout my surgical training and future career.

Though battered and bruised, I made it through training camp and earned a starting position on the freshman football roster. And what better way to officially welcome me to the team than to have a few of the seniors commemorate my fourteenth birthday (October 18). How thoughtful of them. Yes, many of them couldn't wait to find me throughout the school day so they could each *hand deliver* their gifts—*"birthday punches,"* fourteen of them, to be exact, but, thankfully, not to the face. Everything else was fair game, and, thanks to this Neanderthal tradition, for days, I could barely carry my books to class, much less hit a tackling dummy at practice.

This warm welcome aside, being part of a team for the first time in my life was transformative. But predictably, by now, I had bigger dreams for the gridiron. After the season was over, I dedicated the entire off-season, from December to August, to becoming a better football player. Every day after school, I'd work out in the weight room until closing time at 5:00 p.m. If you recall, I have already shared with you that I would cap the evening off with a lengthy study session. That was my daily routine. Each off-season thereafter, I would reinvest the time and effort to becoming the best possible student and football player I could.

By putting in the work, I also proved that physical strength, like intelligence, can be built and coached up. After myriad hours and attempts in the weight room, I finally did it. In June of my freshman year, this fourteen year old became only the second or third football player in KHS history to enter the 1,350-pound club as a freshman. This meant that, for the four core powerlifting exercises, I had successfully lifted the minimally required weight for each, adding up to 1,350 pounds (bench press: 250 pounds; deadlift: 400 pounds; squat: 500 pounds; clean: 200 pounds). When you consider that, only a year earlier, I could barely bench press 150 pounds, for example, this was a monumental achievement for me at the time. The "Kearny Pride 1,350-Pound Club" T-shirt I was awarded became my prized possession. I was tremendously proud of this badge of honor, a reminder of what is possible when you really apply yourself. In the process, between high-calorie protein shakes and my mother's prolific cooking, I had managed to pack on thirty-five pounds of muscle by my sophomore season, earning a starting spot on the varsity team. This was yet another incredible milestone for me. And by the time my senior season rolled around, I tipped the scales at 225 pounds, could bench press 350 pounds, and was named

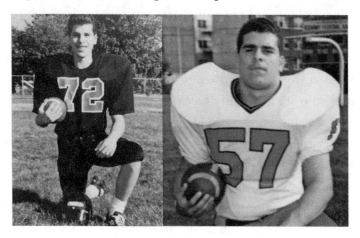

Kearny High School football freshman year (left) and senior year (right)

one of the team captains. This was a far cry from that scrawny 150-pound freshman, nervous, afraid, and desperate to find his place and to make his mark.

Needless to say, no one ever stuffed me into a locker during high school. I had successfully negotiated the tumultuous landscape of locker room antics and alpha male posturing, relatively unscathed. In addition, as an amalgam of being a jock, nerd, loner, and popular kid, on some level, I helped stamp out the clichés attached to these four adolescent prototypes. I was the friendly, happy-go-lucky kid, having earned the unique distinction of simultaneously being the strongest and the smartest (highest GPA and SAT scores) in the entire school. This is no humble brag, just a proud statement of fact on how I was able to seamlessly navigate between these social echelons and to help keep the peace. To say I had come a long way is a definite understatement, but, in the eyes of my coaches and college scouts, I had not come nearly far enough. As much as I hate to admit it, my book smarts never fully translated into football IQ. My speed and agility still left a lot to be desired, and my game stats most certainly didn't pass muster for the next level.

"Who was I kidding anyway?" I wondered, as my dream of having my name called at the NFL draft someday withered away into some obscure recess of my mind. For only a brief moment, the bitter taste of humble pie made this depressing realization very difficult to swallow. But I refused to stay down. I wasn't programmed that way. On to plan B. There was no time to wallow in the mire. My urgency of purpose automatically kicked into high gear, because I knew I had bigger fish to fry. The morale of the story here is that you should never skip dessert when humble pie is on the menu; and be sure to order seconds! Life's about to school you, so take full advantage of the free lesson.

To the extent that I fell short garnering athletic accolades, I made up for in spades with my academic throughput. I was named valedictorian of my senior graduating class, a surreal achievement that cemented my legitimacy as a competitive applicant for the country's most elite universities. With college-application deadlines looming, I was on the verge of making one of the biggest decisions of my entire life, a bold move that could have massive implications for my family and that could drastically alter the course of my future.

"Stay focused and relentless. Repetition is your mission, perfection your obsession, and victory your redemption."

–BRIAN LIMA

CHAPTER 4

HEART OF WAR: COMPLACENCY IS THE ENEMY

*"It's not human nature to be great. It's human nature to survive, to be average and do what you have to do to get by. That is normal. When you have something good happen, it's the special people that can stay focused and keep paying attention to detail, working to get better and not being satisfied with what they have accomplished." –*Nick Saban

I'd say Nick Saban knows a thing or two about success and greatness. Having captured six national titles and built a championship dynasty at the University of Alabama for the ages, he'll go down as one of the best college football coaches of all time. His unprecedented body of work speaks for itself, so, naturally, my ears perk up whenever I hear him share insights about his take on success. I've also grown to appreciate his rather entertaining, matter-of-fact delivery—he tells it like it is and doesn't mince any words. His commentary above

is particularly enlightening. Basically, he's telling us that having success and being great runs counter to our natural tendencies. We're wired for mediocrity, for just getting by, and
for resting on our laurels. Wow! He's calling out complacency.
That's the culprit, the elephant in the room that's holding us all
back. Wait. Is that really all it is?

To get at this question, we begin with the difficult task of
defining "success." Success comes in many forms. It's a relative
term. If you survey a hundred people, you'll get a hundred different definitions and explanations of what success is and why
it matters. Some may offer up a safe, generic statement about
"accomplishing one's goals." Aww, how politically correct of
them! For many, success is all about monetary wealth, power,
or fame. For others, success is not some quantifiable asset or
net-worth calculation. It's not measured by the number of
zeros in your bank account, by hit singles on the Billboard
charts, or by some other worldly construct. They instead view
success in terms of spiritual or physical health, the love of family, and personal relationships. Call it what you will, but, across
all walks of life and, spanning all time, contexts, and venues,
success is a desire we all share. To be, or not to be, successful?
It's not even a question—we all want success, notwithstanding
our individual spin on its meaning. Still with me? Okay, great!
Now, answer me this: what if the second question in that survey was, "If given the option, how often would you like to have
success as you define it—rarely or most of the time?"?

This time, of course, ALL of our responses would be iden-
tical. Regardless of what success means to us, who among us
would not want it most of the time? Or even all of the time? No
budding musician ever dreams of being a "one hit wonder." No
one would want to have a successful business or marriage only

some of the time. The same applies to our health—the more, the better. But that's just it. Success, in its purest, most elemental form, is our common denominator, our universal truth. Not only do we all want it, but also, no matter what floats our boats, we all would ideally have it most of the time. If only we could just snap our fingers and, voila, success on demand.

Therein lies the challenge. Fortuitous or fleeting success is readily attainable by most, but sustained success is a completely different beast. Just ask Nick Saban, Tom Brady, or Michael Jordan. Even a blind squirrel will occasionally find a nut. But reaching the pinnacle of success and staying on top of your game is a ceaseless war of attrition. Guess what's your primary opposition—complacency. Yes, complacency is a dogged adversary that never leaves your side and that fights you every step of the way. The onslaught intensifies, as your success mounts. Many of us remain oblivious to the insidious nature of complacency. Unchecked, this corrosive force will sabotage all aspects of your life, like a metastatic cancer that overruns its helpless host. Everything in your life, from basic needs and overall level of health all the way to the most aspirational endeavors you could envision, is fair game. There's no burying your head in the sand on this one. Sooner or later, it will catch up with you in one way, shape, or form.

"There's a war going on outside, no man is safe from
You can run but you can't hide forever"
–Mobb Deep in "Survival of the Fittest"

The war is waged on multiple fronts, each for as long as you remain committed to that particular brand of success you subscribe to. And the minute you rest on your laurels and kick your feet up, you've *settled* for defeat. At that moment, the war is lost, because you've unwittingly abandoned your urgency of purpose, your moral compass, and your sense of the big picture. You've veered way off course from *the Heart Way*. Maybe you didn't want it badly enough, or maybe you bit off more than you could chew. You may have surrendered to fatigue, or you may have grown increasingly impatient and frustrated with the lack of progress. Perhaps you really hit it out the park so you can afford to coast for a while—eh, wrong answer! Whatever reason or excuse you have for losing your edge and letting your foot off the gas, just know this simple truth: there's always someone hungrier waiting in the wings to claim your spot or to pick up where you left off to take it even higher. In many such instances during the past thirty plus years, that certain someone was often yours truly. Remember: as Babe Ruth said, "it's hard to beat someone who never quits," even if that person is not the smartest or most talented in the room.

That brings me to yet another invaluable life lesson my father imparted long ago, during those kitchen-table chats. Well before Nick Saban let the cat out of the bag, my father had already schooled me on complacency. My father's contempt for complacency was so intense that he could never bring himself to utter it by name, as if so doing would summon its odious humors into our home. Instead, every chance he could get, and especially when I shared my latest academic conquest, he would look me straight in the eyes and issue these fatherly words of caution: *"Ahora no te duermas en los laureles mijo."* Translation: "Okay, son, now don't rest on your laurels." I always nodded in agreement, acknowledging the greater task at hand. Before long, his phrase became permanently etched into my subconsciousness. It was like a flashing neon "DO NOT ENTER" sign to ward off complacency or any other unsavory influence. Don't get me wrong: both he and my mother would get ecstatic upon learning of my achievements, pat me on the back, and heap lots of praise. With their faces beaming with pride and smiling ear to ear, they would love to hear the play-by-play or, better yet, to attend the formal award ceremonies and to witness these milestones firsthand. My father would embarrassingly brag nonstop about me to our relatives and acquaintances, to the point that I'd have to kindly ask him to stop. But as the excitement and celebrations subsided, my dad would dispense his habitual reminders with impeccable timing and delivery. It was a foreboding of the threat complacency posed if I let my guard down and halted my momentum. He knew that I needed to reboot and to get ready for the next mission. I can't thank him enough for this regularly scheduled programming. I needed all the help I could get to meet the challenges that lay ahead.

My father really was the dad that every dad should be. His guiding influence was critical to my development, an uplifting beacon of hope amid a stormy sea of disadvantages and hardships that I was forced to contend with. It saddens me to know that so many kids grow up in single-parent households, desperately lacking that father figure or role model to emulate. Challenging, but supportive, my dad masterfully hardwired a security checkpoint in my brain, barring entry to complacency and not allowing it to get a foothold. You could say he successfully created a monster, the good kind. I was emboldened to make my biggest move yet—I was going to leave home to attend Cornell University, an Ivy League school. This was a massive dream and extremely controversial. No one in my family had ever left home to go to college. Oddly, no one (siblings, cousins, aunts, uncles) EXCEPT my parents were terribly receptive to this harebrained scheme. In a traditional close-knit Latino family, you don't leave home unless you're married and you're going to start a family of your own. Cornell? I was asked repeatedly by extended family about why I wanted to go. "Why can't you just go to a local college, like your brother or cousins did? You want to become a doctor? Who's paying for that schooling? How can you abandon your family and not stay at home to help pay some bills?" From their perspective, these seemed like legitimate questions. At the time, an Ivy League school was something no one in my family even knew or cared about. They had no idea or comprehension of what Cornell was, or the Ivy League, or what opportunities and doors this kind of education could open for me. I might as well have been saying I was going to Wonderland or Oz. But I'll give my parents credit for blindly trusting my judgement. They totally had my back on this one and took a lot of heat from the rest of the family in the process! They said that if I could get a scholarship, I had their blessing. So that's precisely what I had to do, and, thankfully, working my tail off to be valedictorian was enough to get accepted to Cornell University as a Cornell National Scholar on almost a full ride!

You may be wondering how or why I picked Cornell. By today's standards, this part of my story will sound utterly shocking or insane. These days, kids often go on lavish cross-country college tours, visiting many different campuses with their parents. After thoroughly vetting all the pros and cons, they finalize a list of schools to which they'll eventually apply. Contrast that with me, who applied to Cornell sight unseen, never stepping foot on the campus until I moved into my freshman dorm. We could never afford to go away on vacations, period. Day trips to the Jersey Shore or Six Flags, maybe, but frolicking across the picturesque arts quad of some random college campus was definitely not going to make my parents' agenda. As a rising senior in high school, all I knew was that I loved chemistry and that I wanted to fulfill my pre-med classes in college. The notion of being a doctor "sounded cool," and my father's earlier heart trouble got me thinking about that career path ever since. The Internet didn't exist yet, so my primary source of information was a random binder of college rankings in the guidance counselor's office. It was there I learned Cornell was a top-ranked chemistry and pre-med college. My teachers sang its praises, and, with the unique option of "early decision" to boot, I could find out relatively soon if I was accepted. I decided to go for it, and, fortunately, the wonderful news came in December. I didn't need to apply anywhere else or subject myself ever again to the painful process of using the prehistoric typewriter. I had the rest of the school year to mentally prepare for what I just signed up for!

What awaited me at Cornell was a rude awakening. I thought I had it all figured out by now. My study system was automatic and foolproof, or so I had assumed. Chemistry had been my best subject, and, after taking first place in New Jersey's very own "Chemistry Olympics" (yes, this was a thing) for my mesmerizing molecular model of caffeine, how could I not major in chemistry? But what dawned on me in a hurry during freshman orientation was the intimidating realization of just how fierce the competition was going to be at this elite university—the best of the best students from all over the world. Many had gone to very prestigious boarding schools or academies or had studied at some of the nation's best school districts. A number of students I came across had also grad-uated at the top of their classes and managed to rack up huge amounts of AP (advanced placement) credits. Of course, I learned very quickly that unsolicited oversharing of these self-aggrandizements was the customary greeting during freshman orientation, coming right after "Hi, my name is X." After they all had dispensed with the formalities of small talk, this awkward show of dominance became rather unsettling to me. It took me a while to find *regular kids* who were just looking to make new friends and not to obsessively engage in this game of one-upmanship. I elected to keep my rapidly expanding list of insecurities to myself. I had no AP credits to speak of, but I nonchalantly shrugged it off, like it was no big deal. I'll be okay. Right?

Cornell was no joke. Every single day was a challenge, and just doing your best often felt as if it wasn't good enough. It was gut-check time on the regular, as I struggled to keep pace with the geniuses in my midst. Some of the professors were world-renowned in their field, even Nobel laureates, and hearing them lecture was surreal and intimidating. I was a tiny guppy in this vast *frozen* pond of overachievers. Oh, yeah, did I mention Cornell was situated in Ithaca, New York, and brutally cold for about ten months out of the year? Living on west campus, I had to walk uphill in snow to class, completely barefoot—okay, maybe not barefoot. I will say that the cam-pus is a gorges one! Get it? There are lots of gorges in Ithaca. But I digress…

One day early on, as I sat in my General Chemistry class with several hundred of my classmates, the professor, curi-ously, asked for a show of hands from all those interested in becoming doctors. Wouldn't you know it! A sea of hands shot up instantly. "Now look to the left, and look to the right," the professor went on. "One of you won't be here at the end of the semester." Say what? General Chemistry was among the core pre-med requirements, and you'd be hard-pressed to find any medical school willing to accept anything less than an A in that course. But how do you separate the best from the best? I'd come to find out it often entails a harsh weeding-out process. Grading was done on a bell curve, where the mean, or average, was set to a C-. So in order for you to get an A-, or better, you had to perform two standard deviations better than the average student in that class. The "average student"? When I considered that all of the students had themselves been prolific overachievers to justify even being at Cornell, this all seemed ludicrous and unjust.

Gritting my teeth, I knew I had my work cut out for me, and I pressed on. I went about my business preparing in my usual way for the first major chemistry exam. I committed all of the lecture notes to memory, along with the corresponding textbook chapters. I went back through all of the assigned problems until I could do them in my sleep. The day finally came, and I sat down, ready to rip this exam a new one. There was just one minor technicality. I stared in disbelief, as I flipped through the pages of the exam booklet. I couldn't do a single problem. One question read as follows: "Forget the laws of chemistry as you know them. You now reside on planet X where the following principles govern the properties of molecules......" I wanted to barf. We all walked out of that exam in a daze, completely shell-shocked from this traumatic reality check!

Our collective performance on the exam was abysmal. I scored barely one standard deviation above the mean, putting me somewhere in B range, a grade I hadn't seen since junior high school. All things considered, it could've been a lot worse, so I felt somewhat relieved. This was my official introduction to the big leagues and how you weed out the best from the best. The professor had assumed that all of the students, including me, could have effortlessly regurgitated anything from the lecture notes or the textbook. But this ain't Kansas anymore! Rote memorization and pattern recognition were child's play. Sadly, this proved to be too much to overcome for many of the students. They were quick to hit the panic button and folded under pressure. They all had big hopes and dreams, until they had to put in the long hours and tackle tough exams. As time went by, the number of hands raised grew appreciably smaller, and students got weeded out. Some quit, others failed, and some changed majors altogether.

Going to Cornell was a huge gamble for me, and I felt like I had to make it count. Were all the naysayers right? As I struggled to study and to make sense of things, I heard my father's voice in my head: "Work hard, don't rest on your laurels, and nothing comes easy." I was determined more than ever to succeed. I was not about to give up that easily or to face the "I told you so's" from family back home. Complacency with my amateurish approach to studying had lulled me into a false sense of security. This was the wake-up call I needed, and I sprang into action. If I had any chance of salvaging an A in General Chemistry, I was going to have to completely revamp and overhaul my studying tactics. When I received my graded exam back, I scoured through it like a crime-scene investigator, hoping that the postmortem analysis would shed some light on the errors of my ways. After I delved deep into the forensics, it became clear I didn't know the subject as well as I had presumed.

In retracing my steps, I also uncovered what it really meant to be a doctor. To my surprise, the word "doctor" is derived from the Latin word *docere*, meaning to teach or instruct. The young, aspiring physician that I was embraced this concept, and that's when things began to make more sense. The ultimate litmus test for true mastery of a subject is being able to teach it to someone else because you have intimate knowledge and understanding of how the information comprising that subject was formally derived. For example, the classic equation from Einstein's theory of relativity appears so deceptively simple, $E=mc2$. If given the values for "m" and "c," even a high school student could easily calculate what "E" equals. But how this equation was derived and its implications encompass a body of mathematics and science so complex that few people on this planet can barely comprehend it. The point is that things don't just magically appear in textbooks out of the blue, conveniently packaged to spoon-feed the masses. There's a backstory, a methodology for how that information came to be or for how that equation was deduced. A deep understanding of that backstory requires a whole new level of tenacity and inquisitiveness. I brought all my faculties to bear on this novel strategy, and it payed major dividends. Slowly but surely, I methodically inched my way to a final grade of A- in chemistry that first semester. Elated, I felt like I had just cracked the Da Vinci Code and snatched victory from the jaws of defeat.

But I didn't stop there. I couldn't. There was blood in the water, and I couldn't resist the feeding frenzy. After I had slayed the savage beast of introductory General Chemistry, Cornell no longer seemed invincible. I was reinvigorated for the hunt, and even bigger game were lurking on the horizon—Physics, Calculus, Organic Chemistry, Biochemistry, and Physical Chemistry. Suffice it to say, these other goliaths met the same fate. But at what cost? This is the time when the rubber met the road, and I was studying day and night! To minimize distractions, I lived and studied in the same dorm room (Mennen 205) all four years. I figured, "If it ain't broke, don't fix it," so why mess with success? I was a creature of habit anyway, and I had grown very fond of my private little mission control center, complete with glow-in-the-dark star stickers on the ceiling my predecessor had painstakingly arranged into several constellations. And you thought I was a nerd? At times, my parents would express their concerns about my well-being, given all the academic pressures, urging me not to take things too seriously. I reassured them that all was good in the neighborhood and that they should just keep those care packages coming. My stores of rice and beans needed constant replenishment for the newly *Cubanized* white kids on my floor, who couldn't get enough of this tasty brain food.

My parents had created a monster, and there was no turning back. I was in the zone, full throttle. Sleep is a luxury badassery rarely affords! When all was said and done, I graduated *magna cum laude* in chemistry—high honors in one of the toughest majors from one of the world's best colleges. Not bad for the son of poor Cuban immigrants. It gets better. The ultimate cherry on top was getting accepted into medical school, which, in and of itself, was exceedingly difficult. But, somehow, by the grace of God, I had been awarded a dean's full tuition scholarship to one of the top medical schools in the country, Duke University School of Medicine, down in Durham, North Carolina.

I had always been a fan of Duke basketball, having watched New Jersey native Bobby Hurley play for the 1991 and 1992 national championship squads. For whatever reason, I never thought of Duke as place to study, nor could I imagine myself living in North Carolina. That all changed when I looked at the medical school rankings in the *U.S. News & World Report* during the year I was applying. Duke was ranked number three, right after Harvard and Johns Hopkins, and shared with the two an alarmingly low acceptance rate (less than 5 percent). Harvard didn't even offer me an interview, and I was wait-listed at Johns Hopkins. Duke saw something in me that the other two didn't, and, for that, I will be forever grateful! Words alone could never do justice to the joy this amazing news brought to me and my family. Out of thousands of applicants to Duke Medical School, I was among the lucky *one hundred* accepted students entering the first-year class in the fall of 1998. Never in my wildest dreams could I have ever scripted such an amazing opportunity. I was well on my way to fulfill my dream of becoming a doctor.

It goes to show you that where's there's a will, there's a way. We're capable of so much more than we give ourselves credit for, but we're often unwilling to probe the possibilities. As David Goggins aptly summarizes in his motivational masterpiece, *Can't Hurt Me*: "We habitually settle for less than our best; at work, in school, in our relationships, and on the playing field." Whether on an individual basis or at the corporate level, there's always room for improvement. Eking out the highest quality possible requires sustained and meticulous attention to every detail and never settling for the status quo. No one ever said getting to the top is easy. The perilous drive is long and fraught with potholes, speed bumps, traffic jams, and other road blocks impeding our ascension to the Promised Land. I saw too many of my fellow students get complacent along the journey and prematurely pull out of the race.

For all intents and purposes, most of these students had a definite leg up on me. They were from affluent families, attended fancy academies, and had every other imaginable advantage money could buy. So what happened? Why did they fizzle out in college? It seems they likely settled into a state of "complacent mediocrity," as Frank Bruni explains in his book *Where You Go Is Not Who You'll Be.* He sheds further light on the underlying cause for this let down:

> "The homogeneous group of overachievers who make it to Princeton or Yale have, to that point, known only one triumph after another, largely because they've been given extensive preparation to master precisely those tracks that the elite educational track values. There was a stunning fragility to some of them. The parental bubble wrap and the boot camps got them to their one and only goal in lives, 'a top-ranked school.' Once there, they're sort of frozen, adrift."

They succumbed to complacency, pure and simple. They lost their momentum, drive, and purpose. I thankfully snapped out of it and could never let myself get complacent. I remained steadfast. Seeing the bigger picture and keeping my eye on the prize was crucial for me. I had to look at it as a competition with myself, pushing myself to be my very best. You can make your own life, your own greatness, and your own success. Whenever you're faced with a major challenge, project, or assignment, you have a choice to make. You have a choice to skate by or to buckle down, work hard, and stay focused. At the end of the day, that's all you can do—control what you can control and let the chips fall where they may. That's how I've managed to keep my sanity and not wither under the pressure of expectation, internal or external. I realized early on that I was just a constant in the multivariate equation of life. I could control my contribution to the equation, like the "c" in E=mc2, but the final outcome for any given scenario was also going to depend on those other variables. But, taking it a step further, I knew that if I really brought the heat and maximized my contribution, it may very well dwarf the impact of those other variables and have the major say in how things turned out. In this vein, think of complacency as a negative "fudge factor" that fractures your contribution and therefore diminishes your overall role in the end result.

There will be dark times. Invariably, and on more than one occasion, life will knock you on your ass. That's okay. Don't fret. Just get right back up, dust yourself off, and keep moving forward. As the old adage goes, "the beatings will continue until morale improves." You will be either the one who simply gives up or the one who is successful and wins. Being truly resilient means finding solace in that faint, flickering light of hope during the darkest moments of despair, when the full weight of the world is against you yet you defiantly rise to meet the challenge, unfazed. Strive to be like Rocky Balboa in all his final fighting scenes, especially against Clubber Lang (*Rocky III*) and Ivan Drago (*Rocky IV*—my favorite). Get mad, get even, not in a malevolent way, but recycle the pain and disappointment of failures and setbacks into a motivational force, a turbo boost. Become better, stronger, and wiser. When life gives you lemons, take them willingly, say "thank you," and turn them into something amazing! Forget lemonade! That's so passé! How about a novel substrate for renewable clean energy. Instead of going green, we'd all go yellow, and you win a Nobel Prize and save our planet! Catch my drift? Flip negatives into positives and think big when you do so!

But whatever you do, don't ever get complacent. No matter how far you've come or how great you think you are, life will remind you who's boss and will jam a giant piece of humble pie down your throat! I could've gone the other route, but I elected to exercise restraint and keep it clean. Constant motion, growth, and development are the essential vitamins and minerals for our soul. Like the shark that must never cease swimming, we must never cease working on and bettering ourselves. If you're reading this and you've grown complacent, how can you make a change? You know when you've gotten complacent in certain areas of your life. Maybe it's your fitness or your family or your business. If you're at the top of your game, you can tend to slide and rest and think you don't have anything else to learn. This happens to people all the time. If you've already become the best in your industry, you may think you don't have to train or grow any further. Or maybe you just haven't worked out in a different way in years, and you know that it's time to train harder, lose those extra five pounds, and eat healthier. Whatever it is, only you know. Whatever you do, don't become complacent. You're never too cool for school. Complacency is the enemy. To be complacent means to give up, to shrug, and to care less. You're better than that...get after it!

"Elite performance requires countless moments enduring life's toughest torrents."

–BRIAN LIMA

CHAPTER 5

HEART ACT TO FOLLOW: LEARNING FROM THE BEST

"Winners in life have clearly defined, constantly referred to, game plans and purposes. They know where they're going every day, every month, every year. They're objectives range all the way from daily priorities to lifetime goals. And when they're not actively pursuing their goals, they're thinking about them—hard!" –DR. DENIS WAITLEY
(THE PSYCHOLOGY OF WINNING)

Now that we're a few chapters in, we're practically family! Let's retrace our steps to get some perspective on how far our journey together has taken us. We've covered a lot of ground in a short time. We've established that we are each capable of great things, so long as we believe in ourselves and are willing to put in the time, effort, and hard work to make our dreams a reality. We are the true masters of our own destinies and need to simply get out of our own way. With sheer will power and work ethic, we can overcome many of our intellectual and physical shortcomings via *heartificial* intelligence. Finally, we can never afford to settle comfortably into cruise control and rest on our laurels. There's nothing passive about this process, because self-discovery and self-improvement are lifelong endeavors. It's not a means to an end, because, technically speaking, there is no end—"mastery," as Daniel Pink points out in his book *Drive*, "is an Asymptote [a straight line that approaches a curve but that never quite reaches it]…You can approach it. You can home in on it. You can get really, really, really close to it…But, you can never touch it…the joy is in the pursuit more than the realization."

With all that said and done, where does that leave us? Are we now fully equipped to take the world by storm and to reach the pinnacle of success in the field of our choosing? Not so fast. Granted, yes, having all these synergistic elements working together on our behalf already puts us way ahead of the curve, but it does so only to a certain point. You see, at this juncture, we've only been addressing our own internal limitations and how to maximize our innate capabilities. In doing so, we've managed to build a powerful jet engine, its tank brimming with rocket fuel. But there's more to it than that. The engine alone doesn't make the vehicle. I'm no gearhead, but even I know that if you were to put a Ferrari engine in my pickup truck (yes, I drive a pick-up; it's awesome), there's still no way I could successfully negotiate a hairpin turn at high speed. Such a stunt would not be death-*defying* but more like death-*certifying*, and the poor rescue crew would have one hell of a time finding my scattered remains.

The point of my graphic dramatization is that, apart from a Ferrari's powerful engine, there are obviously many other factors and technical refinements that have cemented the Ferrari's place as the standard by which all other sports cars are measured—one of the greatest of all time (G.O.A.T.). These nuances, ranging from aerodynamics to independent suspension, have all been painstakingly optimized to complement the capability of the robust engine. If tasked with building the next best sports car, you'd better believe I'd start with the Ferrari blueprint and learn all I could about the ins and outs of the car's masterful design. It's this process of reverse engineering, of learning the tricks of the trade from the best of the best, that marks the next major formative step of our journey and my personal story.

Had I relied solely on my homegrown diesel engine, it's doubtful I would have gotten into medical school or excelled in my professional surgical career. My father's lessons had stuck, and I could hang with the best of them in college. But good grades alone were not enough. Like it or not, there's, regretfully, some element of truth to the saying, "It's not what you know that matters; it's who you know." I'm not at all implying, or condoning, the practice of career advancement for those less qualified on the basis of powerful friends in high places. But I do acknowledge that you have to finesse and hustle to navigate effectively in any competitive landscape, to learn the ropes, to network with the right people, and to accumulate the requisite experiences to stand out in a crowd of similarly qualified applicants. The right people are the "who" here, the ones who know how to play the game or who have the 4-1-1 on who does play the game. Getting into medical school, especially a top-tier one, is an incomparable "resume arms race" (Lukianoff and Haidt, *The Coddling of the American Mind*), and the race is only getting worse. What you know is not nearly enough in this arena. I often joke that Harvard Medical School didn't even offer me an interview because, aside from my good grades, I wasn't an Olympic gold medalist or world-class concert pianist. In all seriousness, though, life is unfair that way. I suppose it's just human nature, but it's obvious we just can't help ourselves—we love to feel special or important. Everywhere you turn—be it academia, industry, government, or the social scene—there's always some unspoken V.I.P. section enclosed by an invisible velvet rope. To be on that guest list or to even know that section exists, you need to be special. You need to be in that inner circle, or at least know someone inside it that can sneak you in through the back door.

Thanks to a few of my college dorm buddies, the extent of my naivete in this regard came to light early on. Some were from a family of doctors and could obtain extensive "health care experience" with relative ease, logging hours by shadowing their families or their colleagues. They also knew about the importance of other extracurricular activities, such as laboratory or clinical research, to help bolster your application to medical schools. There again, they had connections, direct and indirect, and could readily secure these limited positions. The list goes on and on, and it was expanded even further when I spoke to college seniors that had been accepted to medical schools. Their tips and insights on what worked and what didn't were absolutely priceless. I had stumbled upon my Ferrari archetypes, my examples to emulate, and the keys to the V.I.P. section. By virtue of my incessant scavenging for the inside scoop and reverse-engineering efforts, I amassed a stout portfolio of experiences and avoided an untold number of pitfalls along the way. To be the best, you have to learn from the best. That's the moral of this story. Don't hate the player; hate the game!

Playing the game, as it were, also forced me to get out of my shell in college and to really broaden my horizons. Between my marathon study sessions, I would've been quite content eating my Ritz crackers and playing solitaire in good old Mennen 205. But, alas, the life of a hermit is not entirely compatible with being a go-getter. For nearly all four years of college, I worked in a medicinal plant chemistry laboratory, studying the medicinal properties of tropical plants. For my honors thesis, I discovered the presence of reseveratrol, a known antioxidant, in the tropical vine *Gnetum nodiflorum*—do I have you on the edge of your seat yet? Try this one on for size—I also worked as a T.A. (teaching assistant) in organic chemistry my junior year. This activity forced me to work on my public speaking skills, by giving review lectures to hundreds of students. The toughest cookie to crack, however, was getting my foot in the door to the medical field. The most gaping deficit in my candidacy for medical school was "clinical experience," or lack thereof. Clinical experience was a buzz phrase that was the bane of my existence throughout college. Try as I might, I had a hard time landing any substantive clinical gig. Sure, I could have volunteered as a candy striper at my local hospital, like so many of the other pre-med students. However, I felt that would've hardly been the case cracker for my clinical experience woes. After searching far and wide, I finally found, applied to, and was accepted to a very competitive pre-med summer research program at NYU School of Medicine in Manhattan, between my junior and senior year. Little did I know that this initial exposure to real clinical medicine would prove to be a major defining moment and turning point in my life.

I was fortuitously assigned to shadow one of the general surgery attendings (aka professors). For the uninitiated, a general surgeon is a physician who has completed a five-year residency training program after medical school and who has expertise in trauma and in operating on all of the organs in the abdomen (appendix, gallbladder, colon, liver, pancreas, and the like). General surgery residency is a prerequisite for further subspecialty training in cardiac surgery, plastic surgery, and surgical oncology, to name a few. Each of these "fellowships" entail as many as three years of additional training. So, during residency training in surgery, you start as an intern in your first postgraduate year (PGY) after medical school. You proceed along up the ranks all the way to chief resident as PGY-5 and beyond, during fellowship training. This nomenclature will be important later, when I recount other personal vignettes, such as my going all the way to PGY-10, the longest track in all of medical-surgical training, to become a full-fledged heart surgeon, subspecializing in heart transplants and mechanical heart devices. More on that later...

Now that we've got those technical details out of the way, we can pick up where we left off with my story. As part of my shadowing experience at NYU, I was immersed in the crazy, intense militaristic culture of surgical residency. It felt like being in the movie *Full Metal Jacket* on a daily basis, where the attendings and the senior and chief residents were the drill sergeants, the hospital ward and operating rooms our boot camp, and the rest of us different iterations of Private Pyle. As with any stereotypical hierarchy, you know what rolls downhill, and this was no exception. Believe it or not, I loved it. It instantly brought me back to my old high school football days, with our head coach barking at us constantly. NYU was, at the time, considered one of the more prestigious, yet harsh, training programs in the country, ruled with an iron fist by the world famous chairman Dr. Frank Spencer, a beloved giant in the field of heart surgery. On his passion for the field of surgery, Dr. Spencer was quoted as saying, "Unique to surgery is the creative use of one's hands to cure or improve human disease." That says it all!

Unexpectedly, I was infused with a sense of comradery and passion with my assigned team that seemed familiar and comforting at the same time. I felt like I was part of something important, for the greater good. Then, out of the blue, it happened. The definitive, mind-blowing experience came when I was asked to scrub in and watch an actual operation. It's a moment that I'll never forget, because, at that instant, it struck me like a lightning bolt—the ultimate epiphany! "This is it! This is what I want to do! I don't care how long it takes or how grueling it will be, but I want to become a surgeon!" There was just something magical about watching someone manually removing a life-threatening tumor with such incredible poise, dexterity, and precision that struck a chord with me. I was completely awestruck. The surgeon I was shadowing, Dr. Stuart Marcus, was very encouraging, and I, in turn, made a favorable impression on him by program's end. It turned out that he had attended Duke Medical School, and he was gracious enough to write me a glowing letter of recommendation. Watching and learning from the best in action had once again tremendously benefitted my career path.

That fall, I returned to Cornell for my senior year as a changed man with a rejuvenated clarity of purpose. Before, I wanted to attend medical school so I could become a generic doctor. Now, as I explicitly shared on my medical school applications, it was specifically all about becoming a surgeon. The difference now, of course, was that I could convincingly back up my reasoning because of the transformative experience I had just had at NYU. Duke heard my calling loud and clear, and I anxiously awaited the official launch of my medical career in Durham, North Carolina. The question now was how to spend my last semester at Cornell before graduation. A good number of my classmates came down with a severe case of *senioritis*. I'd hear them crack jokes like, "What do you call the person who graduates last in his medical school class? A doctor!" Under the gripping spell of this virulent contagion, they whimsically blew off the rest of the year, took courses in wine tasting, and went skinny-dipping in the gorges. I know; it does sound like a lot of fun. Believe me, I love having fun just as much as the next guy (I swear, I really do). But the game was far from over. I needed to keep my head in the game and not waste any precious time. Thanks to Papa Lima, I was fully immunized against senioritis, so I instead elected to take full advantage of the remaining time I had at this storied institution. I took courses that would prepare me for the rigors of medical school, including physiology and neurobiology. By now, you know the drill. If I thought college was tough, I was about to tangle with a murderers' row of ninety-nine intellectual mutants, all top-notch students handpicked from the most prestigious universities in the country. It included about twenty from Harvard, twenty from Yale, twenty from Duke, a handful from Cornell (including myself), and the list goes on. I couldn't sit idly by and wait for the onslaught. I had to be proactive and to ready myself for the big game.

Believe it or not, at Duke, we would be graded on an

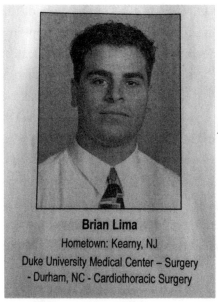

First day of medical school at Duke, 1998. This was right after my audition for The Jersey Shore—*kidding!*

Brian Lima
Hometown: Kearny, NJ
Duke University Medical Center – Surgery
- Durham, NC - Cardiothoracic Surgery

HONORS, PASS, FAIL system. That sounds better than typical A–F grading in some respects, but to get an H (HONORS) in a course, your final average score had to be within the top 10 percent–20 percent of this class of all-stars. I kid you not, but, in some of those first-year courses, the thresholds for H range were as high as 93 percent! This was the case for gross anatomy, a highly vaunted course, where everyone went full-beast mode to secure an H. On the basis of my prior intel, I was well aware of the importance of getting as many Hs as possible—that's how you got elected into AOA (the Alpha Omega Alpha Honor Medical Society), the Phi Beta Kappa of medical school. Many competitive residency programs, especially within surgery, would not even consider your application if you failed to reach AOA status.

But wait; there's more! As I'll go into greater detail later in the book, the Duke General Surgery program was among the most prestigious and selective in the country, one of the big four, as we used to call them then: Duke, Johns Hopkins, Massachusetts General Hospital (the MGH—Man's Greatest Hospital), and Brigham & Women's (the Brigham)—the latter two hospitals are Harvard Medical School's primary teaching hospitals. Duke's surgery residency program director was Dr. Ted Pappas, a luminary in the field of hepatobiliary surgery, and a famous graduate of the Brigham's surgical program. To make a long story short, if you didn't spend a month as Dr. Pappas' subintern (sub-I) in your fourth year of medical school and secure his blessing on paper (letter of recommendation), you had a snow ball's chance in hell of getting into Duke, the Brigham, or any of the other upper-echelon surgery programs in the country. Keep in mind that these surgery programs have only about seven slots a year, so you really had to be something special to get in. And the hits just kept coming.

In yet another astonishing example of *it's not what you know but who you know* in action, about ten of us (yes, I was wise to the game by this point—Mama didn't raise no fool) in the first-year medical school class reserved our sub-I slot with Dr. Pappas more than three years in advance, within a couple of months of starting medical school. How crazy is that? I can still recall how baffled his administrative assistant was when I called. Our class of neurotic gunners had taken their obsessive compulsions to a whole new level. She couldn't believe this many of us were signing up so far in advance. By the time I caught wind of this madness and jumped on the bandwagon with my frantic call, I was lucky there were any available openings on Dr. Pappas schedule to accommodate another student on his team. You snooze, you lose, and it became crystal clear, right out of the gates, that my first-year comrades were going to keep me on my toes for the foreseeable future. To keep pace with this thundering herd of GOATs, I had to rise to the occasion and step up my game. They forced me to get better by making me acclimate to this higher level of intensity and performance.

The bottom line is that just when you think you've peaked, or maxed out, on your capabilities, you're still probably only scratching the surface of your true potential. Don't just take it from me. Take it from David Goggins, a former Navy SEAL and record-breaking endurance athlete:

> "Even when we feel like we've reached our absolute limit, we still have 60 percent more to give...Once you know that to be true, it's simply a matter of stretching your pain tolerance, letting go of your identity, and all your self-limiting stories, so you can get to 60 percent, then 80 percent and beyond without giving up. I call this The 40% Rule,...if you follow it, you will unlock your mind to new levels of performance and excellence in sports and in life."

A case in point was my tried-and-true study approach. I thought I had perfected my system, but I was wrong. It, too, needed an upgrade, because the sheer volume of information tested on each exam was several orders of magnitude greater than anything I had encountered in college. In fact, thanks to Duke's unique curriculum, we were covering twice the amount of material in our first year than any other medical school in the country. How can that be, you're wondering? Well, traditional medical school curriculums consist of two years of classroom instruction, with courses like gross anatomy and pathology, followed by two years of clinical rotations and electives in all the various medical specialties. Duke had decided that, instead of having two years of classroom instruction, it would condense all of it into an eleven-month hellacious first year, freeing up the third year to engage in independent research.

My first year of medical school was an absolute blur, as you might imagine. We would be in class approximately eight hours a day, and major exams were given almost weekly, typically on Mondays. I became a studying machine, and weekends amounted to over forty-eight hours of heavy mental lifting. To handle the volume of material, I instituted a digital upgrade to my handwritten cheat-sheet technique. Because I could type much faster than writing by hand, this switch alone dramatically improved my efficiency. Okay, I know you're thinking it, so just say it out loud—"work smarter not harder," blah blah. Fine, I know I poopooed it before, but, just this one time, I'm okay with that saying. Moving on, one of the perks of being a medical student was that we were each given our very own laptop. I put this handy dandy device to good use, typing out my cheat-sheet notes in very small font (eight points) in a format of two columns per page. With two columns, it was easier to keep my place while scanning over each line of text. I remember condensing our entire neurobiology textbook (coincidentally, the same book I had used during my senior year at Cornell) into twenty pages of this typed microscribing.

I weathered this yearlong blitzkrieg, getting HONORS in almost every single course, including gross anatomy. I don't know how I did it, but I can tell you it's the closest I'd ever come to burning out. The crazy thing is that I'm pretty sure I was nowhere near the smartest student in the class. In fact, I'm willing to bet that if we were to have taken an IQ test (which, thankfully, we weren't required to do), I would've scored in the bottom five out of these one hundred cyborg savants. Of course, I may be wrong, and we'll never know for sure. But one thing is for certain—I worked harder than the other ninety-nine students. There's no question in my mind: with sheer willpower, I beat that info into my skull until I retained it, even if took a heck of a lot longer than the rest of the class. I wanted it more than anyone else. That is the key! If you truly want to be successful when you pursue something you are passionate about, you MUST want it more than anyone else. That's the way of the GOAT, no matter the field. You can't talk about it; you have to be about it! I live it; I breathe it every day. It is part of me and my heart.

We were allotted only a month-long respite, before gearing up for round two. My brain was mush, and I was running on fumes. But there's never any rest for the weary. What lay ahead for the second year of medical school was a completely new adventure, where we would be graded on the basis of our clinical performance on an actual medical team, spanning the gamut of medical specialties. Over the course of eight weeks on surgery, then internal medicine, ob-gyn, pediatrics, and so on, we would be subjected to the steepest learning curve any of us had ever faced. It's one thing to know you have a test in a week and you can prepare for what will likely be asked on that exam. It's another thing altogether to "get pimped" (to get asked tough clinical questions by senior level residents or attendings) on the fly, at random hours of the night while on call and sleep deprived, on rounds, or in the actual operating room during a surgical procedure. Gone were the days of being able to study from the comfort of your own home, conveniently around your precious schedule. The new mantra that would forevermore govern all of our lives was "eat when you can, sleep when you can, and leave when you can." You studied whenever and wherever you could. Let's just say success in the classroom doesn't always translate into success on the clinical wards. We all had to adapt and overcome. You either knew the answer(s) or not, and your ego had to be okay with your knowledge deficits being aired out in a public forum.

With the mounting pressure of getting that precious H ever looming, it was easy to get visibly flustered and emotional during these relentless interrogations. Such loss of composure was a big red flag, an unshakeable sign of weakness. There's no crying in surgery—yes, the surgery rotation was particularly egregious in this regard. Smelling blood in the water only egged the interrogators on, and these humiliating proceedings could get pretty ugly and painfully drag on. The struggle was real, and only the strong survived in this shark tank. The key, I found, was to stay cool, calm, and levelheaded, even when you didn't know the answer. Somehow, as it had worked in football practice years earlier, this was a useful damage-control tactic. Years down the line, I overheard one of our notorious surgical attendings share this with another resident: "It's no fun yelling at Lima. The more I scream, the calmer he gets!"

He was absolutely right. Never let them see you sweat, baby. But, obviously, just stoically getting by would not amount to a winning strategy if I whiffed on most of the questions. At the end of the day, it's a matter of life and death, so you have to know what you're doing. How are you supposed to explain away not getting an H in surgery on your surgery residency application? Chances are you may have blown it, no doubt because there were several other applicants that aced their surgery clerkships. I wasn't having that, so I took a Navy SEAL approach to this new challenge—assault by air, land, and sea.

As an aside, when in doubt, you can't go wrong with this strategy. Having sought the counsel of savvy third-year and fourth-year medical students, the Ferraris of their respective classes, I got the lowdown on how to pummel these clinical rotations.

Their first piece of advice was to channel my inner chameleon and do my best to blend in seamlessly with the culture of each medical team I was assigned to—"When in Rome, do as the Romans do." If they stay late, you stay late, and so on and so forth. The second pearl of wisdom they imparted was to make myself useful above all else, by having a firm grasp of the three As of physician success: be affable, available, and able. That all seemed like common sense, but it was much easier said than done. Medical students often got a bad rap for needing a lot of hand-holding on clinical teams, having to be explicitly told where and how to be helpful or when to go eat lunch, when to go home, and so forth. They felt lost and disoriented in this callous, fast-paced jungle of patient care. Many were also perceived as lazy—say, for not being present, perhaps goofing off somewhere, or studying in the medical student lounge, or racking (sleeping) in the call room. They failed to realize that you will never be given the benefit of the doubt in such a cutthroat environment. Your absence, to most, will be attributable to the worst-case scenario, especially in the sardonic world of surgical training. The prevailing creed uttered repeatedly during medical school and residency was, "Trust no one, expect sabotage."

Many medical students, then and now, still don't get the picture and predictably fall into the same trap. Rather than rolling up their sleeves and proactively helping their clinical team, they sit around passively, waiting to be assigned their next task, with their head buried in a book or worse yet, with their eyes staring at their smartphones. As such, rather than becoming active, contributing members of the team, they're relegated to irrelevant bystanders, shepherded from activity to activity, just passing the time until being dismissed for the day. I'm sure you would agree that such a pedestrian performance is not exactly "HONORS worthy." It should therefore come as no surprise to them when they see a PASS on their transcripts for their time served on that clerkship.

To be the best, you quickly learn that "just enough" is way too little. No exceptions. You have to go above and beyond, as did the great ones before you. If you don't know who the GOATs in your field are and all about their "secret sauce," then it behooves you to find out. Everything. STAT! By "STAT," I mean right away, at once, or immediately, if not sooner—not *Some Time At your Trivial* convenience! Reverse-engineer their success into a set of habits and behaviors that you closely mimic or duplicate. In subsequent chapters, I'll go into greater detail on how I adopted this strategy at each successive stage of my career progression. And just to be clear: this strategy applies to ALL fields, not just health care. In many respects, the hospital is no different than any other place of business imaginable. There are always piles of work that need to get done. If there really, truly is absolutely nothing left to be done, then first, I don't believe you, and, second, do yourself a favor and look busy anyway.

On the clinical wards, there was always some scut work to help with, some radiology result to hunt down, or some other task the team needed to get done. I didn't need to be asked to help because I was already on it, like a regular Johnny-on-the-spot! My aim was to become the medical student that all teams wanted on their service, and I made the most of it on every service I was assigned. While I certainly wasn't the GOAT, I successfully achieved HONORS in most of my clerkships, including surgery, where I solidified my intentions to pursue this career track. The stage was now set for the next chapter, not only for this book but also in my lifelong journey chasing greatness!

PART TWO

IN *HEART* PURSUIT: BLOOD, SWEAT, & YEARS

"You rise, you fall, you're down then you rise again
What don't kill you'll make you more strong."
–Metallica in "Broken, Beat & Scarred"

"Own your past, cherish the present, and never bank on the future."

–Brian Lima

CHAPTER 6

FOR THE MOST *HEART*, GRAVITAS IS A MUST

"I gravitate towards gravitas."—MORGAN FREEMAN

"Why are you getting wrapped up in petty no-difference crap rather than the kinds of issues and actions that are going to move mountains, that are going to authentically engage you with real progress, real accomplishment, and real purpose? You can't keep responding in ordinary ways if you are truly out to live an extraordinary life."—GARY JOHN BISHOP

Morgan Freeman's iconic voice is one of a kind, perhaps the best ever in Hollywood. Whether he's playing God or a convict (*Shawshank Redemption*) or simply narrating a wildlife documentary, we've all grown quite enamored with his powerful voice. His soothing tone never misses the mark, simultaneously conveying his depth of character, wisdom, and authority. If he's telling me to make a left on Waze, I'm making a left, no questions asked. Most would agree that if you looked up "gravitas" in the dictionary, his picture would, or should, be included as the quintessential personification of this ancient virtue. Whatever gravitas is, he's got it.

That said, I must admit that "gravitas" is not entirely a straightforward word to define. It's one of those "I know it when I see it" type of phenomena. We've all witnessed it at some point or another. Apart from Morgan Freeman, other examples abound. You could've seen "gravitas" when you've heard one of Martin Luther King Jr.'s moving speeches, a lecture by one of your tenured college professors, a State of the Union address delivered by President (insert your favorite), or Marlon Brando as Don Corleone in *The Godfather*. The last example may be debatable, given he's playing a mobster, but you know what I'm getting at—the acting is second to none. The common denominator here is that these individuals exude an impactful "I'm the real deal" aura that captivates our attention, respect, and even admiration.

Gravitas originated as one of the four principal virtues of ancient Roman society, along with pietas, dignitas, and virtus. It connotes seriousness, commitment, depth of character, and purpose. Isaac Newton, the father of calculus and physics, thought so highly of this virtue that he named "gravity" after it! In today's business world, it's synonymous with having an *executive presence,* that extraordinary combination of looking, sounding, and acting like the undeniable leader that everyone wants to follow. In my world of heart surgery, it's the consistent ability to calmly and expeditiously deliver live-saving technical mastery in the face of chaos and impending death for someone on your operating room table. A more formal definition of gravitas would encompass the following traits:

"There are six elements of gravitas critical to leadership: grace under fire, decisiveness, emotional intelligence and the ability to read a room, integrity and authenticity [people don't like fakes], a vision that inspires others, and a stellar reputation."
—Sylvia Ann Hewlett

That's a mouthful. For the longest time, "gravitas" was just another funny-sounding Latin word I had occasionally encountered during my preparation for the SAT exam. I had a vague sense of its meaning, just enough to correctly identify its synonyms or antonyms on a test question. Beyond that, it bore no meaning in my life or relevance in my methodically crafted battle plan for success. That all changed, however, during my first year of medical school. If you recall, Duke's innovative curriculum included a third year completely devoted to independent research, in whatever area of medicine or science you selected. Naturally, like every other calculated move in this epic chess match, the "ideal" experience would have to deliver a major competitive upside and blow that of my opponents, I mean, classmates, out of the water. I know, it sounds harsh, but that's really how it went down, because that's how most of my contemporaries were approaching the matter. By now, you know I'm not going to sugarcoat anything—past, present, or future. I call it like I see it…

It had to be this way because of the competitive nature of many of the residency programs we were all after. There are many more graduating medical students than there are residency slots every year. The bottleneck that exists for the most sought-after specialties at the most prestigious institutions was, and remains, alarmingly narrow. Depending on the specialty—such as neurosurgery, orthopedics, ophthalmology, plastic surgery, and general surgery—each program may offer only have a handful (one or two, even) of positions every year. The nice thing about this year of research was that you could strategically structure an experience perfectly suited to your intended specialty and really set yourself apart from other applicants. So, to get the biggest bang for your buck, you would zero in on a particular laboratory or research mentor that fulfilled some basic criteria. For starters, your research mentor needed to be a "heavy hitter," with great renown in your field of interest. Leveraging your mentor's sphere of influence could make all the difference in landing that highly coveted residency slot. But having the big name reference was not enough. There's always more to it than that. You also had to be productive—your experience needed to generate evidence of your academic throughput in the form of research publications in medical-scientific journals and in presentations at national meetings—"publish or perish," as they say. That meant your mentor had better have a prolific track record with ongoing research efforts, churning out publications on an industrial scale. Get your name on a few of those bad boys and you're good to go—wham, bam. Simple, right?

Easy, tiger. Notice that I failed to mention anything at all about having a *genuine passion* or interest in the research endeavor as a prerequisite. In reality, this should have been the most important factor. That other stuff is important, but it is far outweighed by how meaningful the work would be to you and within the grand scheme of things. Was the research going to make a difference, change the practice of medicine, help our understanding of some deadly disease, or help me grow as a scientist or a clinical investigator? B-O-R-I-N-G! None of those questions were factoring into my misguided selection process at the time. Instead, I had distilled my decision down to the purely ulterior motive of maximizing my competitiveness for residency programs. I had lost my way. As William Damon describes in his book *The Path to Purpose*, I had abandoned that "stable and generalized intention to accomplish something that is at the same time meaningful to the self and consequential for the world beyond the self."

So there I was, in the thick of it, robotically self-absorbed, prospecting, making my rounds, and scheduling meetings with different high-profile scientists at Duke to find my golden goose. Like any typical high-strung gunner, I felt like I was behind the eight ball, because many of my overachiever classmates already had racked up multiple publications on their CV (curriculum vitae, aka resume). My college research had never amounted to a publication, so I felt a bit self-conscious having comparatively fewer lines on my CV. In retrospect, that may have further clouded my judgement. I was so caught up in the CV arms race that I had lost sight of my true purpose and had become misaligned with my moral compass. Does that sound vaguely familiar? Perhaps such gross imprudence is what partly drove the corrupt practices uncovered in the recent college-admissions scandal. It's possible, but, in my case, there's no doubt I had again wandered off *the Heart Way*.

When you're stuck on the hamster wheel, as I was, the world can get away from you in the blink of an eye. All you can focus on is running, so you lose sight of the forest for the trees. I was totally oblivious about my wayward descent until one of the shrewd scientists I sat down with tactfully called me out and set me straight. I must have been two or three questions in when he abruptly cut to the chase and brought me back down to Earth. My line of questioning about his research

must have been an embarrassingly dead giveaway for someone preoccupied with quantity, not quality, as I was. This was
no run-of-the-mill scientist, if there is such a thing. With his
MD and PhD (double doctorate), he was a physician-scientist,
a true "triple threat," who split his time taking care of patients,
running his research lab, and teaching and training medical
students and residents. Such a rare breed was not to be trifled
with, and he saw right through my BS. He had had gravitas for
days. Like most physician-scientists of his caliber, he intentionally chose not to disseminate his work in piecemeal fashion, with multiple insignificant publications. He insisted on
grand works of high quality, telling more of the "whole story"
and therefore warranting publication in the most impactful
of scientific literature. Think of him as the Dos Equis guy—he
didn't publish often, but when he did, it was big-time stuff!
Most of his work was published in major medical journals,
like the *New England Journal of Medicine* or the *Journal of
Clinical Investigation*. Each publication constituted a massive
contribution to the medical field, helping countless physicians
and patients all over the world. He was unwavering in staying
true to himself and to his purpose. His work had to matter—
that's gravitas!

I had a lot to learn. He helped me realize that I had gone
about this the wrong way. As a complete neophyte in this
regard, I had been blinded by misguided ambition for stack-
ing my CV. Here I was, like some lovesick puppy dog, content with any morsel of research so long as it was published
somewhere, anywhere, even in *The Throw Away Journal of
Medical Obscurity*, if such toilet reading existed. I finally saw
the light and realized how far off track I had gone. I forcibly
extricated myself from the hamster wheel, rededicated myself

to my purpose, and did a lot of soul searching. I vowed that my work needed to matter. too. It needed to have meaning and a tangible connection to something greater than myself, and it needed to help advance the field of medicine. Of all the things I had studied in medical school, what had really moved me and sparked my interest?

The answer to that question became crystal clear a short time thereafter, during my immunology class. I was spellbound by the science of transplant immunology and how organ transplantation had become the gold-standard treatment for several end-stage diseases. Reading about the history of transplantation and key milestones was equally riveting. The first kidney transplant was performed by Dr. Joseph Murray at the Brigham in 1954. A few years later, in 1967, Dr. Christiaan Barnard performed the world's first heart transplant in Cape Town, South Africa. It got me thinking: "How cool would that be—to become a transplant surgeon?" It seemed like the perfect marriage between amazing science and amazing surgery. Hmm…more on that later.

Meanwhile, it was deeply troubling for me to learn that thousands of people die every year waiting for an organ transplant. The critical shortage of available donor organs to save the exponentially growing number of people who need them is only part of the problem. The immunosuppressive regimens required to prevent rejection in those fortunate enough to receive organ transplants not only have many dangerous side effects but also can't prevent "chronic rejection." That is to say, over time, the immune system can unavoidably overwhelm the transplanted organ, necessitating a redo transplant. Widely acknowledged as the Achilles' heel of transplantation, this erosive process is the immune system's version of Chinese water torture, unfolding over the course of years and evading clinical detection until the horse is out of the barn.

I had finally found my cause. I sincerely wanted to join the fight against transplant rejection and to help solve the organ-shortage crisis. I haven't looked back since. Why? A huge reason comes from what happened next—I learned about the pioneering work of Dr. David H. Sachs, a renowned immunologist and the director of the world's premiere transplant laboratory, the Transplantation Biology Research Center (TBRC) of the MGH at Harvard Medical School. You could fill an entire book with all of his seminal contributions to the field of transplant immunology, but a book still wouldn't do his contributions justice. Among his many volumes of "greatest hits," you can find his landmark studies in the areas of immune *tolerance* (duping the immune system into accepting a transplanted organ without using antirejection drugs) and *xenotransplantation* (transplanting organs across different species, from pig to baboon, for instance). Fancy medical jargon aside, few scientists have done more to advance the science of transplantation or to unravel the mysteries of rejection. Not to get into too much technical detail, but there was no better mentor or laboratory in the world better suited or equipped to pursue my passion for this space. And that's precisely why I fell out of my chair when he replied to my email inquiry about working with him for my research year! It's a good thing I didn't break my neck, because I was in store for an incredible adventure.

By following my passion and abandoning petty self-serving pursuits, I found that everything was falling into place. Dr. Sachs kindly agreed to be my research preceptor and helped me complete a grant proposal. I received a prestigious fellowship from the Sarnoff Cardiovascular Research Foundation to fund my year of research with Dr. Sachs at the TBRC. Under the tutelage of this exemplar of gravitas, I learned the nuances of research, what good science was all about, and what it meant to make a real dent in the field of medicine. Even now, when I mentor students and residents with their research projects and manuscripts, much of what I share is derived from what I gleaned from Dr. Sachs. You see, with gravitas, the halo effect of positivity can span many degrees of separation from its original source. Sure, when I do surgery, I'm directly impacting and saving that individual patient, but when I can help advance the field of medicine or help inspire future leaders in health care, my positive scope of influence is magnified several times over. It brings me that much closer to making our world a better place. That's what it's all about! It should never be just about you!

This point is worth elaborating on further. Almost more significant than what gravitas is are all the things gravitas is not—i.e., those physical, behavioral, and verbal cues to the outside world that you're anything but someone to take seriously, ill-qualified to be entrusted with important matters or positions of authority. These days, a classic example that comes to mind is compulsively looking at your phone during an important work meeting. Even if you're just checking work emails (wink, wink), the optics of this inconsiderate behavior are off-putting to your colleagues and superiors. It sends the message that while you may be physically present, you're not fully engaged in the meeting and more concerned about your Facebook newsfeed. Remember it's human nature to assume the worst, so no one's going to give you the benefit of the doubt in these instances.

What really grinds my gears is the rampant practice of using the word "like" repeatedly as a filler when speaking. It's like nails on the chalkboard. If it, like, takes you, like, at least three-to-four "likes" to, like, make your point, then, like, you probably, like, lost your intended audience by, like, the second "like"! It's this and other annoying speech trends, such as "upspeak" and "vocal fry," popularized and continually propagated by so-called social media influencers, that can really derail the efficacy of your communication in any professional setting. So don't be discounted because of the way you deliver your message. Speak with gravitas! Spare us the agony!

You also need to act and to look the part. Clearly, appearances matter. You must be aware of how you are perceived by others. Some call this emotional intelligence or self-awareness, but, no matter what you call it, it's another level of intelligence that you must nurture if you want to develop gravitas. Increasingly, however, and especially in professional venues, time-honored formalities in body language and attire are giving way to more casual, dare I say, downright flippant, tendencies. In my job, gravitas is imperative when speaking with other doctors or with patients and their families. It's a vital facet of bedside manner. Patients and their families are trusting me with their lives. If I exuded anything but gravitas, they would not be so receptive to what I have to say. Can you imagine what it would look like if I showed up to speak to your loved one about a major surgery while looking as if I had just rolled out of a ditch somewhere, a disheveled mess in wrinkled scrubs? It'd be like a scene right out of a GEICO commercial, where you'd be begging for a "second opinion" right after I blurted, "But I just saved 15 percent on my car insurance." Some people may find this level of attention to appearance silly, but it goes back to the idea that appearances do matter. Whatever situation you're in, you must be intentional about presenting yourself in a way that is appropriate for that setting.

It's perhaps a bit of an extreme example to cite as a point of reference, but I can vividly recall how tightly wound I became as a surgery resident in the hallowed halls of Duke University Medical Center. I had survived Duke Medical School and my sub-I with Dr. Pappas, earning an Alpha Omega Alpha distinction for being among the top students of my graduating medical school class. As one of the lucky seven to "match" (get accepted) at Duke for the seven-year general surgery residency program, I was about to officially start doctoring. Normally, general surgery requires only five years, but Duke requires an additional two years dedicated to research, typically undertaken in years three and four. You see, Duke was not interested in training just surgeons. Duke was, and is, all about training the future leaders in the field of surgery, surgeons with gravitas.

Duke's program, a paragon of prestige, rigid hierarchy, and meticulous attention to detail, was akin to running a marathon at a sprinter's pace, while simultaneously drinking out of a fire hose. It had long been rumored to be the most demanding and stressful surgery training program in the country. Adding to its mystique was the infamous "greater than 100 percent divorce rate" among its trainees—according to legend, many of the Duke surgery residents got divorced more than once during their training. When queried by applicants to the program, the residents' scripted response was of the "can't confirm nor deny" variety. Loose lips sink ships, but this reputed statistic was more part of the folklore of the program than actual fact. My divorce, for example, didn't happen until a couple years *after* I finished. But, seriously, it's still one of the first questions I'm asked by other surgeons when they find out I trained at Duke—"Was the divorce rate really that high?"

The intense culture of the program was firmly entrenched and established by the legendary Dr. David Sabiston, chair of surgery, father of heart bypass surgery, and author of what many deemed the bible of surgery, *Sabiston Textbook of Surgery*, currently in its twentieth edition. Incidentally, Dr. Sabiston was a contemporary of Dr. Frank Spencer, who, as I mentioned in the last chapter, was the chairman of surgery at NYU. They trained together at the great Johns Hopkins Hospital decades earlier, served in the military together, and were essentially cut from the same cloth. Now in its ninth edition, their authoritative treatise *Sabiston and Spencer Surgery of the Chest* was required reading for anyone in the field of cardiothoracic surgery.

During Dr. Sabiston's thirty year tenure (1964–1994) and beyond, Duke graduated innumerable luminaries that would eventually lead surgical departments throughout the country. Many of these giants in surgery had also done their heart surgery training at Duke, rounding out their "decade with Dave," another oft-quoted nod to the rigors of this storied program. As you walked down the main corridor of the surgery department, leading up to a bust of Dr. Sabiston, you could see signed portraits of all the previous graduates hanging on the *wall of fame*, a true "Who's Who" in the world of surgery.

Living up to this legacy of excellence was a tall order for its trainees. Simply stated, perfection was the expectation in and out of the operating room. Any deviation from this expectation, no matter how seemingly minute, would be promptly lambasted. Whenever any of your boneheaded blunders came to light, it wasn't uncommon for you to be chastised with, "And that's why it's a ten-year program!" On the other hand, positive feedback for a job well done was seldom, if ever, granted, because it seemed silly and disingenuous to get a pat on the back for something you were supposed to do anyway. And we wholeheartedly bought into this philosophy. All of us checked our egos at the door. We always knew where we stood, and delusions of grandeur were as scarce as a good night's sleep.

Sleep? What's that? It was a rare commodity in those days. Regardless of how sleep-deprived we were, we *always* had to appear clean-cut, well-groomed, dressed in formal attire (shirt, tie, crisp white lab coat), in full command of all the "data" (lab and test results, vital signs, and the like) for every patient under our care, and ready to tackle the litany of tasks continually being added to our to-do list. Life became all about checklists and the seemingly unwinnable game of checking off every empty checkbox. Just when you thought you had conquered the day's tasks, your chief resident would inevitably assign several more on evening rounds—a handful of things to get done before you could call it a day. The typical day started at roughly 4:00 a.m., and it was only 10 p.m.— plenty of time left before quitting time. And heaven help you if you were caught outside of the O.R. in your comfy *pajamas*, aka scrubs. That could easily get you fired on the spot.

Dr. Hilliard Seigler, one of the most senior Duke master surgeons, said it best: "There's an intensity of work here. There's a level of sophistication and accomplishment that is not present in most surgery training programs…And for many, many years we have maintained that level of intensity… it's been one of the hallmarks of our success." The bottom line was that we always had to "look the part," to be presentable and professional for our patients, our staff, and our faculty. This imbued us all with a true sense of pride, purpose, and zeal for this exacting science we were fortunate enough to pursue. We rose to the occasion. We learned to BE at our best even when we really *felt* like we were at our worst. Your moment may come when you least expect it, so we always had to be ready! Life happens, not on your schedule, or conveniently during "regular business hours." The same applies to sickness and disease, traumas—you name it. Our duty was to seize these moments without hesitation, morning, noon, or night, calmly facing each crisis the same way every time, with precision, skill, and intentionality. Faltering was not an option. I cherish those days, because they made me the person and the surgeon I am today. Unpleasant as it was, this was the foundation necessary for the development of my gravitas. How could it not? It was essentially force fed to us every day as part of our steady diet. To this day, I have Dr. Sabiston's signed portrait hung up on the wall behind my office desk, symbolically "looking over my shoulder" and constantly holding me accountable.

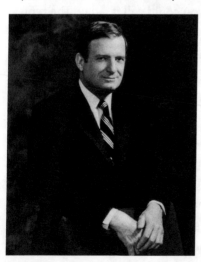

Dr. David C. Sabiston, Chairman of Surgery at Duke University Medical Center (1964–1994), gravitas personified.

But times have changed. Our mainstream society has grown accustomed to instant gratification, constantly searching for the next "life hack" or "quick fix" (David Goggins, *Can't Hurt Me*). Our tech-savvy youth, who spend countless hours staring at screens, are bombarded with a host of non-traditional role models, courtesy of social media. From reality TV stars to Instagram models, these glamorized replacements for the role models of old (doctors, teachers, lawyers, and the like) are direct threats to the viability of gravitas. Indeed, the currency for success today is measured more by the number of followers or "likes" you have than the length of your resume or the degrees on your wall.

"A popular culture celebrating quick results and showy achievements has displaced the traditional values of reflection and contemplation that once stood as the moral north star of human development and education. Instant mass communication transmits tales of highly envied people who have taken shortcuts to fame and fortune to every child with access to computers and televisions." —WILLIAM DAMON

By all accounts, short of maybe the military and professional sports, the days of tough love and accountability are long gone. As mentors or educators, we are forbidden to openly critique those under our wing. Anything deemed even remotely offensive can get you "written up," reported to HR, or subject to dismissal, depending on the subjective severity of the violation. We have therefore become risk-averse auto-pilots on the path of least resistance. Positive reinforcement is the name of the game, and, win or lose, all participants walk away with a trophy.

This makes you wonder about our so-called right to the "freedom of speech." Technically speaking, yes, you have the right to share your opinion or voice your discontent, without any fear of criminal prosecution. The court of public opinion is another matter altogether. Carelessly speaking your mind—in whatever forum, private or professional—can land you in some pretty hot water, even if you had the best of intentions. There now exists a political minefield in virtually every nook and cranny of our lives. If you're lucky, your less-than-perfect word selection may fall on deaf ears and not ruffle any feathers, but that happens rarely. Chances are that whatever you say and however you say it, someone, somewhere, will take offense to it. This is the world we live in. To err on the side of caution, you're more often than not better off keeping your words to yourself instead of "thinking before you speak."

We've all become so fearfully obsessed with being *politically correct* (PC) that we walk on eggshells around our trainees and they run amok, emerging ill-prepared to meet future challenges and the harsh realities of life. As eloquently described in the book *The Coddling of the American Mind,* authors Lukianoff and Haidt elaborate on the emerging culture of "safetyism" and how today's youth have a greater proclivity for irrational thought patterns, typified in anxiety and depression disorders, such as catastrophizing and negative filtering:

> "[The] culture of safetyism is based on a fundamental misunderstanding of human nature...that allows the concept of 'safety' to creep so far that it equates emotional discomfort with physical danger...that encourages people to systematically protect one another from

the very experiences embedded in daily life that they need in order to become strong and healthy."

Come on! If I were to have equated emotional discomfort with physical danger, I would've never made it out of junior high, much less out of the trials and tribulations of getting my butt handed to me on a daily basis during a decade of surgical training. It's hard to fathom how or why we've let things get so out of hand. The ship may or may not have already sailed on halting the progression of these troubling cultural trends. The societal forces at play are incalculable, intertwined, and likely irrevocable. But gravitas is not an extinct virtue. At least it doesn't need to be so long as we can get it off the endangered species list. It's just infinitely more difficult to engender in a society held hostage by the hypnotic grip of social media and other confounding variables. As individuals, we each have a say in the matter. The onus is on us to pull ourselves up by our bootstraps and to fight the good fight. We must snap out of it and strive to reclaim gravitas for ourselves and for those under our stewardship. That said, we may, realistically, never acquire that one-of-a-kind, smooth, sage Morgan Freeman voice, but it's certainly worth a try. I'm game. Are you?

We'll close out this chapter with some parting words of caution. The struggle is real, and we live in some crazy times. How you present yourself in public is more important today than ever before in history. The Information Age has ushered in a tremendous amount of technologic advancements and has enabled the globalization of industries, economies, and cultures. But the unanticipated downside of the Internet and social media has been the eradication of any semblance of privacy we once took for granted. Now, more than ever, the

negative ramifications of lapses in gravitas can be quite catastrophic. Everything we do today is under a microscope. "Big
Brother" is always watching, so assume that any indiscretion
or misstep—past, present, or future—can be used against you
and can lead to your demise. Your career could be ruined in
an instant, if you are captured on video or in a picture doing
something questionable. The media abounds with stories of
politicians, professional athletes, and celebrities who have
ruined their reputations through social media. No amount
of money, fame, or political clout can shield you from the
ever-watchful eye of the public, nor the consequences of your
misdeeds and wrongdoings.

As C. S. Lewis once said, "Integrity is doing the right thing
even when no one is watching." The same can be said for gravitas. Why not strive for excellence 100 percent of the time?

There are many conflicts and stressful situations that come
up day to day. Taking the moral high road and keeping your
composure are not always easy, but they are necessary for
you to succeed in whatever you want to do in life. There's no
way around that. Always take the high road, no matter what
WAZE is telling you. No short cuts allowed. The HEART WAY
will never lead you astray.

"Don't become a victim of circumstance. Insist on being the victor of happenstance."

–BRIAN LIMA

CHAPTER 7

KICKSTART MY *HEART:* EMPOWERED BY AMBITION

"Without ambition one starts nothing. Without work one finishes nothing. The prize will not be sent to you. You have to win it."—RALPH WALDO EMERSON

"You can't measure what's inside a man's heart."—JOE ROGAN

Had enough of my nostalgic trips down memory lane, yet? It's a rhetorical question, but if I had to guess your answer, I'm going with a "just about." At any rate, we're *just about* in the home stretch, and our time together will soon come to an end. A few more of my corny stories to make some heartfelt points, and you'll be much the wiser—at least I hope! So please indulge me another brief visit to a simpler, happier time in my youth. It was the early 1980s, and VCRs still didn't exist. Attention millennials and iGen: VCRs were videocassette recorders that preceded DVD players. Forget about DVR or Netflix—you might as well have been talking about time travel. The only way to watch a new episode of your favorite show was to actually watch the episode live, at the precise time it came on, together with family or friends. I know this sounds crazy and unbearably inconvenient by today's standards. Without any technologic workaround, such tough sledding was immutable. No pause-rewind-fast-forward buttons, to speak of...You and everyone else gathered around the TV had to sit through all the commercial interruptions. You actually had to pay attention to the show and, yes, even to one another, which wasn't too difficult. It's not like you had other distractions, say a smartphone you were constantly staring at, Googling those actors in the show to see what else they've been in, what their estimated net worth was, or what sort of drama they'd been caught up in on TMZ. Smartphones, the Internet, and social media were several years away from their debut. These were the good old days, when people did a much better job of living in the moment rather than feverishly capturing every special event with their smartphones to show off—I mean to share—on social media. It's when "living your best life" had true meaning. But that's enough reminiscing for now.

This sort of good old-fashioned quality time with your loved ones is indeed a rarity these days—a true shame, if you ask me, because the youth of today have no idea what they're missing out on. Maybe that's a topic for another book, likely by another author, but it's the backdrop for the introduction of my next 1980s relic—"turbo boost." One of those shows we all gathered around to watch every week with great anticipation was *Knight Rider*, a series starring Michael Hasselhoff as the crime-fighting do-gooder Michael Knight and his souped-up, blacked-out Pontiac Firebird named KITT (Knight Industries Two Thousand). The show's theme song alone was killer and way ahead of its time, a sort of early predecessor of techno music with a catchy tempo. And KITT was no ordinary muscle car. It was a high-tech, bullet-proof, and fully automated fortress on wheels that could speak, drive itself, and, best of all—it had *turbo boost*. No matter how thick of a jam Michael was in, KITT was always there to the rescue. Hope was never lost, and no obstacle or foe was too difficult to overcome. All Michael had to do was press the "turbo boost" button to activate KITT's rocket boosters. Suddenly, they would be launched out of harm's way, speeding away at a breakneck 200 miles an hour and on to face next week's villain.

Fast-forward almost twenty years to my senior year in college, when I was interviewing for medical school admission. During my visit at the renowned Johns Hopkins School of Medicine, one of my interviewers shared an unusual observation about my application. I'll never forget what he said, because it caught me off guard, so much so that I recall myself kindly asking him to repeat himself, because I wasn't sure I heard him correctly. He said, "Ahem, it appears you were shot out of a cannon!" Huh? He went on to explain that this was, in fact, a compliment, an acknowledgement about how far I'd come and how much I'd accomplished, considering where I had started. It was pretty clear to anyone reviewing my application that I was hell-bent on achievement and that, no matter how disadvantaged I was, I would work harder than anybody else to get the job done. I thanked him for the compliment and said something like, "I see what you mean. It's like I used *turbo boost* or something." Clearly not amused by my *Knight Rider* reference, he awkwardly nodded in agreement and dove right into the meat of the interview. So much for small talk.

What he called being "shot out of a cannon" I was calling "turbo boost," and, for our purposes, I'll be referring to it as *ambition*! Yes, the propulsive power of ambition has been one of the most impactful forces in my life. It gave me the courage to swing for the fences and to chase this crazy dream of becoming a heart surgeon. Without ambition, I'd be back in Jersey, playing it safe close to home and feeling sorry for myself. I would have proven all of my critics and naysayers right. "You'll never become a doctor." "It's too hard to get into medical school. Even if you do, you could never afford it." "Don't become a surgeon! The training is so many years, so rigorous. You'll burn out for sure! What if you get sued?! It's too risky! Blah blah blah blah…."

Ambition is the antithesis of complacency, that little voice in your head that says, "Ignore them. It's all just white noise. You're in the driver's seat, and you haven't reached your final destination. There's way more to do! Go big, or go home!" And, regardless of your shortcomings or how uneven the playing field is, ambition is the consummate equalizer. It's being able to withstand life's biggest misfortunes and to bounce back from them that makes all the difference. Your eagerness to move ahead contributes more to your success than natural talent or being born with a silver spoon. That's because there's no ceiling to ambition or limit to the amount of cap space available for your will to win. And that's precisely what Joe Rogan meant when he said, "You can't measure what's in a man's heart." Ambition is the ultimate motivational force, the spark that lights the fire in your belly and that keeps stoking the flames as you trudge along your quest. In your darkest moments, when things seem hopeless and you're on the verge of calling it quits, ambition can save the day!

Time and time again, ambition has come through for me in the clutch, just like KITT's turbo boost did for the Knight Rider on so many nail-biting episodes. Not merely "a strong desire to be successful," as the term is generically defined in any dictionary, ambition is more of a multidimensional force of nature with many cohesive elements. It's a combination of eagerness, optimism, growth mindset, grit, tenacity, and passion. When properly channeled, it can manifest profoundly beneficial effects in your life, even in the most trying of circumstances. The key, of course, is knowing which buttons to push so you can readily access your turbo boost when you need it the most. But, like any powerful weapon, ambition must also be wielded responsibly, not blindly or with any malicious intent. In the wrong hands, ambition can become a WMD (weapon of mass destruction), serving only self-destructive or Machiavellian agendas. Over the course of this chapter, we'll peel away the layers of this enigmatic force of nature. We'll decipher how and when to apply it in your own life. In the process, I'll throw in a few germane caveats and personal vignettes geared towards keeping you on the straight and narrow. The rest will be up to you. But understand that, as with many other themes presented in this book, ambition won't come easy, and you'll have to work at it. A lot!

Let's begin with the basic premise that, within the armamentarium of motivational tactics and coping strategies, ambition is your very own Swiss army knife on steroids, a space age turbo booster tricked out with a host of other handy amenities. Each is ideally suited to meet very specific challenges that invariably come up along your quest for greatness. Depending on the nature of the dilemma at hand, you may just need a good pep talk from your internal cheerleader to combat your negative self-talk. Maybe the situation calls for your automatic sound filter to drown out the cacophony of your critics and the "advice" from your doubters. The dual-phase amnesiac-pacifier modality kicks in to neutralize the deleterious effects of mistakes and setbacks. You won't be so quick to talk yourself out of greatness at the first hint of any trouble. No, you'll keep your head in the game long after most have given up. And if you're really in a pickle and desperately need a lifeline, well, that's when you whip out the big guns and turbo boost the hell out of Dodge.

Those are all reasons why having this multipurpose tool is so essential. You must never leave home without it. For one, ambition is so empowering, because it enables you to over-come the primary hurdle to success: self-doubt. Nothing sabotages more talented people with limitless potential than self-doubt. This insecurity will paralyze you with fear and will leave you in a perpetual state of inertia. If you do muster the courage to take your leap of faith and to chase your dreams, crippling self-doubt may also curtail your efforts along the way. Whenever I feel self-doubt creeping into my subcon-sciousness, I have a go-to mindset switch that my father drilled into me decades ago. It starts with asking myself a very simple question: "If other people, mere mortals just like me, could accomplish that feat, why can't I?" In an instant, all of my anxiety, reluctance, fear, and doubts begin to fade away. Everyone puts their pants on one leg at a time. No one is enti-tled to or predestined for success. Some may have a leg up, but victory is earned, not bestowed.

My father masterfully implanted the seed of ambition in my brain. I don't know how he did it, but I'm so glad he did.

After he gave me that initial push, I've been running on auto-pilot ever since. Ambition gains considerable momentum of its own, after you overcome that initial inertia, which is the most difficult step. He always maintained that there was nothing magical about achieving success. If other folks can do it, you can do it, too. Once you get over that psychological hurdle and fully embrace the reality that "no one is special," the sky's the limit! Look out, because you're well on your way and only you can stop you.

It's probably obvious to you by now but I happen to be a huge sports fan. One of the things that always gets under my skin is hearing these commentators, pundits, or columnists completely dissect an elite athlete's performance. Some of them, having never played any sport and lacking any remote semblance of athleticism anywhere in their body, feel completely obliged to hammer away mercilessly at this flaw or that one, at one "terrible performance" or another. Many command a huge following on social media, with hordes of other armchair quarterbacks chiming in, to give their two cents on the matter, as well. Opinions are like smartphones, and everyone has to have one, down to the least qualified, least experienced, or least athletic person in the room or out there in cyberspace.

On some level, I can empathize with the plight of these professional athletes. It's hard to imagine what it must feel like to hear or to see your name being trashed on mass media, but all of us are subject to the callous scrutiny of the public, just on a much smaller scale. Surely it's a heck of a lot easier to stomach these verbal assaults when you command a multimillion dollar salary and lucrative commercial endorsement deals, but that doesn't completely assuage the toll such scrutiny takes on your psyche. Only the true greats of any sport can shut out all this noise and can focus on delivering their best, game in game out. How do they do it?

Not to take anything away from professional athletes, but many have the ample time and resources to invest in an entourage of individuals that help insulate them from the critiques, such as sports psychologists, therapists, and trainers. With the best personnel money can buy, they have all the time in the world to focus solely on bettering their game. Theirs is a fantasy existence few of us could comprehend—their livelihood is playing a sport they love, really well. The rest of us, on the other hand, are not that lucky. We have to tough out our mundane existence and to figure things out for ourselves along the way. If we're lucky and true to ourselves, we also dedicate our livelihood to something we love. But if and when we stumble, we don't have a posse of yes-men there to help us pick up the pieces. It's our cross to bear.

But there is one thing we all have in common, whether we're household names in the sports world or just regular Joes carving out an honest living. We all know that criticism, judgements, and envy all come with the territory. It's the price you pay for daring to stick your neck out and to do something extraordinary. Knowing the source and the impetus for this trash talk is half the battle. That alone attenuates its potency. Those who tried and failed or never tried at all may not be too keen on seeing you fulfill your dreams. These embittered souls have nothing better to do except to project their own insecurities by criticizing the efforts of others. They often lacked the courage, skill, or ambition to be in the vulnerable position of a high-risk, high-reward venture. I've quoted him previously, but, in this department, Dr. Waitley keeps dropping "hashtag truths" on us:

"For many people—the thousands of Losers in daily life—getting through the day is their goal and as a result, they generate just enough energy and initiative to get through the day...having no goals of their own, they sit in a semi-stupor night after night with tunnel vision and watch TV actors and actresses enjoying themselves earning money, pursuing *their* careers and *their* goals."

Ambition means not only ignoring the blatant naysayers and trolls in your midst but also spotting those well-wishers secretly rooting for your downfall. These "wolves in sheep's clothing" volunteer lots of advice you don't ask for, with intentions that, beneath the surface, are a bit suspect. Many, especially those within your own family or circle of close friends, may not even appreciate the biased lens through which they see the world or the shadow it casts on their supposed words of wisdom. A lot of their counsel tends to be very disproportionately "gloom and doom"—that's always a red flag to me. Unless you're proposing something objectively terrible or illegal, those who truly love and care for you should throw in some positive feedback or words of affirmation—like maybe a, "Wow! That sounds pretty tough, but good for you for going for it. I've got your back.". Anything short of that likely means that whatever they're feeding you, it may not be in your best interest, after all. At the heart of it could be some bitterness, envy, selfishness, or even trepidation between the lines—the pursuit of your goal could mean having less of you in their lives or becoming more of a priority than their relationship with you.

Lord knows, I had my share of people close to me who told me my dream was too hard, would take too long, or would not be worth the trouble and stress. This is where things can get pretty tricky and outright treacherous. Discerning which advice is genuinely well-intended or "coming from a good place" is not entirely straightforward. You always have to consider the source of the advice and to take most of it with a grain of salt. Getting a truly unbiased opinion may require a good bit of effort and going well beyond your inner circle to those without any real skin in the game.

And let's face it: if you need to be talked into chasing your dream, then maybe you're not cut out for it to begin with and should reconsider your options. For it to really mean something and to have any chance of success, then your objective or your dream must be so special that you simply can't envision a future doing anything else but that very thing! It keeps you up at night and becomes a pervasive influence in your life, your thoughts, and motivations, leaving little room, at times, for other competing priorities or personal obligations—family and friends. This dream needs almost to be your "precious" obsession, as the Ring was for Sméagol in *Lord of the Rings*. We'll cover that in greater detail in the subsequent chapter.

But, as an example, I'm often asked by medical students or general surgery residents about the "pros and cons" of a career in heart surgery or if I recommended it as a viable career option. My typical response is, "If you need me to convince you, then heart surgery is probably not right for you." It's all or nothing, like the binary operating system of computers that registers only zeroes and ones. You either can't stop thinking about how badly you want it and can't possibly conceive an alternate future for yourself, or you don't—there's no in-between or half-assing allowed. Just as you can't be a "little pregnant," you either are or are not 100 percent committed to this quest. My mind was already made up. No one had to convince me to become a heart surgeon, but countless people along the way attempted to talk me out of it. That's what ambition is all about—identifying a goal, a special goal, and going all in to fulfill it! If it were easy, everyone would do it. That's what makes it special. Visualize. Actualize. Repeat. Never give up!

Ambition equips you with the fortitude and the resilience to continue chasing that faint light at the end of the tunnel. Ambition will carry you through the hard times, and trust me: there will be dark days. There'll be days that bring you to your knees in anguish, when you have to squint your eyes as hard as you can to barely make out that faint light. Life is unfair, and bad things happen to good people more often than we care to admit. If you don't entirely agree with this statement, then brace yourself for impact, because it's only a matter of time. I'm not advocating for living life in the negative but for always being prepared for the worst-case scenario. As the witches in Shakespeare's *Macbeth* anticipated, "Something wicked this way comes." It's coming when you least expect it, and you'll be forced to count your losses, one way or another.

I say this only because I wish someone had told me sooner. Maybe I would have been better equipped to face the impending tragedy of my mother's deadly fight with colon cancer. It came when I had least expected it, at arguably the most inconvenient and crucial time of my young medical career. It happened during my fourth year of medical school, only one week into my critical sub-internship with Dr. Ted Pappas. You may remember, from Chapter 5, that I had signed up for this month-long clerkship three years in advance and that it would be a decisive factor in my candidacy for surgical residency. Dr. Pappas was the program director of the Duke surgical residency program and had trained at Harvard Medical School's world-class Brigham program, so his seal of approval was a must. It all had come down to this, my audition for entry into the world's elite surgical stage. There I was, in the thick of it, pulling out all the stops and weathering this grueling experience as if my life depended on it. Then came a random call from my sister, in the middle of the day. It's not that we weren't close, but we generally only spoke on occasion, and everyone in my family knew that this was "the month" when I'd be out of pocket.

I remember seeing her incoming call on my phone and getting an eerie vibe, as if something horrible had happened. For years now, things on the home front had been relatively stable and uneventful. My parents were in good health and had moved to Miami, or "the Cuba That Never Was," as I often thought of it. They made the big move after my dad retired from the pigment factory, after over thirty years of hard labor. This had always been his dream for as long as I could remember, and he had poured every penny of his savings into finally purchasing a humble little abode. I was happy to see them thriving in their little tropical paradise, close to their native land and along with many other of our relatives. True to form, this "mama's boy" stayed extremely close to both of my parents throughout and spoke with my mother almost every night on the phone. She was my person, by far and away the closest human to me in the world. From my dad, I got mostly tough love, but, from her, the love was more of the "touchy feely" variety. My brother also seemed to be well-adjusted to Miami and settled into his new home routine. My sister was married, with two beautiful daughters, and had stayed behind in New Jersey with her family. They had carved out a nice suburban life for themselves in Cedar Grove, New Jersey, and I visited them a few times a year during the holidays.

When the call came from my sister, I knew my mother was visiting them in New Jersey and getting some quality time in with her grandbabies. I was in between surgeries, rushing to do God knows what, and quickly ducked into an empty call room to answer the phone. That's when my sister dropped the megaton nuclear bomb on me: out of the blue, my mother had undergone an emergency surgery for a bowel obstruction caused by a large tumor in her colon. The tumor was surgically removed, but because there was spread to adjacent lymph nodes, her colon cancer was considered "advanced." CANCER?! She would need to undergo several months of chemotherapy for any chance of cure. I knew the survival outlook all too well, and it was not very promising. At the time, only about forty percent of advanced colon cancer patients survived five years. She was only sixty two years old.

My whole world came crashing down. I never saw this coming, having just spoken with her a day or two prior. She seemed fine. But was she, really? Maybe there had been something brewing, but I had been so caught up in myself and my own little world that I had neglected to ask, or I had overlooked any subtle hints. I was beside myself with fear, guilt, panic, and anxiety: "How could this happen? I can't believe I'm not there for her! What the hell do I do now? I'm going to have to leave, ASAP. There's no choice. If this means I'm out of contention for one of the premiere surgery programs, so be it! It just wasn't meant to be." I was ready to throw in the towel.

I don't know how I kept it together, but I was finally able to talk to my mom by phone, as she came to from the anesthesia. She sounded pretty groggy, and I did my best to reassure her that everything was going to be okay and that I'd be heading up to see her in short order. My words must have roused her from her semicomatose state. "No, no!" she exclaimed. She wasn't having any of that! Insisting that she would be fine, she was more worried about my blowing my chance with Dr. Pappas than that she was facing a deadly cancer and having to recover from a major operation. For years now, I had been obsessively talking up this clerkship, and she knew, just as well as I did, what was at stake. But, at the end of the day, what's right is right. Come hell or high water, nothing was keeping me from seeing my mother! I had already planned on coming up for fall break in three weeks, right after finishing my time on Dr. Pappas's service. I figured I could easily just change my flight, and so I did.

This was the scare of a lifetime for me, and I was really shaken up. Most of us never think something like cancer or an untimely death can ever affect us or anyone close to us. They're just horrible things you read about or see depicted in a *Lifetime* movie. I had taken her for granted, my sweet and selfless mom, the most important and closest person to me in my entire life. I totally lost it when I saw her, not only because we came damn near losing her but also because I knew now that her days on this Earth were numbered. I wasn't going to make the same mistake twice, so I had be sure I made the most of the remaining time we had with her. I didn't know if I had it in me anymore to push forward on this crazy quest. But cancer notwithstanding, my mother's nurturing maternal instincts were still firing on all cylinders. As per usual, most of the time was spent with her comforting me, rather than the other way around. She made me promise her that I wouldn't give up, because I had come too far.

I vowed to keep my promise. After spending a week with

her, I returned to Duke to finish out my sub-I with Dr. Pappas. Thanks to the fall break, I was able to tack on an additional week to his service, thereby fulfilling my entire four-week obligation. I gave it everything I had, and I successfully earned a spot at Duke as one of the seven selected for the general surgical residency program—the only one out of my graduating Duke Medical School class! Had it not been for my mother's selfless love and encouragement, it's implausible to believe I would've somehow powered through that traumatic experience. She was my turbo boost, and her memory remains a prevailing source of inspiration in my bleakest and most challenging times.

About three years later, on December 21, 2004, my mother lost her battle with colon cancer, a few days after her sixty-fifth birthday. The cancer had returned with a vengeance, inflicting a horribly painful erosion into her lower spine. This required an extensive regimen of chemotherapy and radiation that decimated her body, leaving her an emaciated and fragile shadow of her former self. My sister shouldered all the burden of being my mother's caretaker during her final months. My father couldn't afford health insurance to cover my mother's expenses, and, logistically speaking, he had to stay put in Miami to look after my brother. On a measly resident's salary, I also couldn't afford to help the situation in any way. The guilt and helplessness I felt as a result tore me up inside. My parents were therefore forced to live apart, and because my mother's passing occurred suddenly, neither I nor my father was there to comfort her in her final moments. My father, always this unflappable pillar of strength who had never shed a tear, wept uncontrollably, like a child. He was never the same.

He was completely devastated and inconsolable in his

grief-stricken state. In the years that followed my mother's death, things really unraveled. It was as if my mother had been the magical glue holding our family together. My father's health progressively deteriorated, eventually to the point of advanced dementia, heart failure, and emphysema. For a man who never smoked a day in his life to develop emphysema is pretty rare and likely attributable to the toxic fumes he was exposed to all those years in the pigment factory. That's life for you, where no good deed goes unpunished. With his ailing health and mental capacity, my father couldn't continue the upkeep of the house, nor could he continue its mortgage payments. Financially powerless against this economic crisis, I had no choice but to grin and bear the inevitable debacle of my father's dream home. As it went into foreclosure, he transitioned into the care of a skilled nursing care facility to live out the rest of his days. To endure the rigors of my ongoing surgical training, I had to suppress and compartmentalize my grief and despondency over these awful developments. Somehow, I stoically pressed on.

After all of their years of tireless sacrifice and hard work, it's impossible to imagine a more tragic or unjust ending to my parents' story. They didn't deserve to go out like that, and I refuse to accept it as the finale to the Lima story. Their lifelong struggle and commitment to their family will not be in vain. Despite harboring a huge amount of guilt and resentment about how all of this transpired, I still owe it to them and to myself to make good on my promises. I pay down this massive debt of gratitude by systematically converting these negative feelings into a positive, empowering force to keep me on pace. Honoring my parent's legacy has become one of my primary life missions, the turbo boost that has continued to sustain me during all of those gut-check moments when I'm on the verge of admitting defeat. This is what pushes my buttons and what activates ambition when the going gets tough, and I need it the most. It allows me to continue reaching for the stars, as I envision their smiling faces looking down proudly on what their son has become.

Now that I've finished spilling my guts, it's your turn. What pushes your buttons? What do you tell yourself in those trying moments when you've reached your wit's end? How do you muster the strength to go on? Maybe it's also a memory, an inspiring moment or person that can instantaneously rev up your engine and propel you forward towards the finish line. Maybe your source of ambition and inspiration is the belief in a "higher power." I myself, along with about three-quarters of the world's population, can certainly attest to the tremendous impact that religious faith has in influencing one's course of action. I'm, by no means, a Bible-thumping religious fanatic, but my faith in God has been a constant throughout my life. For as long as I can remember, I've prayed my little prayer to God before every major challenge, test, operation—you name it:

> "Lord, I'm faced with a major, major, major challenge. It's because of You that I've been able to come out on top. I hope that, as in the past, You will grant me the guidance, perseverance, and ability to do the best I possibly can, to think things through clearly, to not get frustrated, and to maintain positivity. All of my success I owe to You. Without You, I would be nowhere. I thank You, and I love You for everything You've done for me. I'm eternally grateful! Amen"

I can't provide you literal proof of His divine efficacy, but, anecdotally, deep down in my heart, there's no question that God has blessed every facet of my life several times over and has steadily guided me through thick and thin. But, even for my agnostic-atheist friends out there, this source of ambition doesn't necessarily have to be derived from the worship of deities. It could be a cause, a movement, or a political ideology you wholeheartedly subscribe to that drives your ambitious plans.

The bottom line is that whatever pushes your buttons, be sure you're intimately aware of what those triggers are, and, more important, USE THEM, OFTEN! Use ambition! Let it embolden and impassion you to unapologetically grab the proverbial bull by the horns and swing for the fences. Allow it to work as a force of good in your life. And whatever that dream is that tickles your fancy or floats your boat, go after it, with all your heart! In the process, always take the high road. Operate in a strictly Machiavelli-free zone. Ambition must be rooted in positivity. Your aspirations for greatness should be well-intentioned, and should never come at the expense of others' misfortune. Eradicate from your vernacular and from your mind the ridiculous phrase, "Don't forget the little people." There are no little people. There's just people. Everyone deserves to be treated with dignity and respect. And lastly, it should never be about money! I became a heart surgeon because I was genuinely passionate about it, about saving lives, not about the monetary compensation that accompanies over a decade of rigorous training. Money comes and goes, and no matter how much of it you have, it alone will never be truly fulfilling.

Follow these rules, and the fruits of your labor shall be

plentiful, in due time. Don't get discouraged along the way. You will be tested, repeatedly. Be ambitious. Be patient and persistent, confident but not arrogant. Stay calm, remain positive, and never forget where you came from. Trust in the process, trust in yourself, and trust that everything will work out for the best. As my dear mother used to always say to me, "Lo que sucede, conviene"—everything happens for a reason. Just do your part! You've got this!

"Avoid the ABCDs of FAILURE: Accuse, Blame, Criticize, and Defer. It's on YOU!"

–BRIAN LIMA

CHAPTER 8

TILL DEATH WITH MY *HEART*: ALL IN OR NO WIN

"It's hard to compete endlessly because there's always more to compete with when you get there."—Neil Pasricha, author of *The Happiness Equation*

"Mastery—of sports, music, business—requires effort (difficult, painful, excruciating, all-consuming effort) over a long time (not a week, or month, but a decade)."
—Daniel H. Pink, author of *DRIVE: The Surprising Truth About What Motivates Us*

Have you ever witnessed someone doing something so mind-blowingly stupendous that you wondered if that person might be an extraterrestrial or a more highly evolved species of human? A *Homo* **superion**, instead of a *Homo* **sapiens**, perhaps? The first example that comes to mind for me is Michael "Air" Jordan's signature "flight" in the 1987 NBA slam dunk contest, when he glided to the basket all the way from the free throw line. It still gives me chills every time I see that clip, because it's as if he's defying the laws of physics as we know them. For the longest time, I, along with every other kid in the neighborhood (and probably the entire world), would routinely attempt taking *Jordanesque* flights during pickup games—tongue out and everything. We'd either come crashing back down to earth, well short of the basket, or we'd have the ball embarrassingly swatted into the bleachers. It didn't matter. We all wanted to "Be like Mike," and we couldn't stop trying, because we all now believed we could fly. Jordan's unbelievable spectacle of superhuman athleticism also inspired the "Jumpman" logo by Nike, one of the most iconic emblems ever created in sportswear. Many of us can recite the statistics about all of MJ's championship rings, MVP awards, and the like. His transcendent dominance in the sport of basketball knows no equal, and, in fact, most would readily concede he's the greatest athlete of all time, in any sport, period. To this day, you'll still hear people refer to someone as "the Michael Jordan" of this or that, to emphasize the mastery that individual has attained, relative to his or her counterparts.

That Jordan didn't make the cut when he first tried out for his high school varsity team makes his legacy that much more legendary. He wasn't born "Air" Jordan. He made himself into the greatest basketball player the world has ever seen! According to Tim S. Grover, his long-time trainer and the author of the book *Relentless: From Good to Great to Unstoppable*, MJ was the ultimate "Cleaner, the most intense and driven competitor imaginable." No matter the scope of the problem or what goes wrong, a "Cleaner," as Grover defines it, will reliably and single-handedly "clean" up the mess and get the job done. For Jordan, this translated into an insatiable drive not only to be the best but also to redefine the sport of basketball itself. In the moments immediately following any of his six NBA championships, while his teammates and coaches were still dousing one another in celebratory champagne, Jordan would already be quietly fixated about going for next year's trophy. This thirst for perfection was all-consuming and superseded every other aspect of his life. Grover goes on to describe the extremes to which a true "Cleaner's" relentless approach to excellence will go:

> "The drive to close the gap between near-perfect and perfect is the difference between great and unstoppable. You never shake the uneasy feeling that you can't ever be satisfied with your results; you always believe you could have done better, and you stop at nothing to prove it. Is it an ideal way to live? I don't know. It's not easy, that's for sure. You hope your family and friends ultimately understand. They might not. Your whole life is essentially dedicated to one goal, to the exclusion of everything else...You have to be committed to saying, 'I'm doing this, I'll give up whatever I have to up so I can do this, I don't care what anyone thinks, and if there are consequences that affect the other parts of my life, I'll deal with them when I have to.'"

Sorry; I know this is a long passage, but it poignantly illustrates an important point. It's a summation of what being ALL IN is all about! It may sound a bit too extreme for some of you, but, depending on the scope of your dream, there may be no way around it, especially if we're referring to something that's your true "calling." It's all in or no win, as I've said before, pure and simple. We're not talking about mere hobbies or leisure activities. Not all ambitious plans are created equal, nor do they call for such excessive levels of dedication or overt fanaticism on par with MJ's tenacity. They may not be as grandiose as wanting to be the best athlete that ever walked the Earth. But chances are, if it's really your calling—i.e., something truly meaningful, bigger than just you, and genuinely well-intended—your quest is not going to be a walk in the park. And please keep in mind that "a purpose can be noble without being 'heroic' or requiring daring, life-endangering adventures," as William Damon explains in his book *The Path to Purpose*. "Noble purposes may also be found in the day-to-day fabric of ordinary existence," such as a being the best possible parent to your kids or being the best possible teacher for your students. These ordinary people doing ordinary things, as my parents did for me, are the unsung heroes of our society, the *Michael Jordans* of everyday life. They give everything of themselves, willingly sacrificing their own wants and needs in the service of their calling, without any fanfare or big payday, purely out of the kindness of their hearts and the devotion to their causes. No man is an island unto himself, and you can't have an alpha without a beta, or an omega. That is to say, the individual succeeds if and only when his or her "pack" succeeds. All members of the pack each serve a vitally important function, even if their purpose is to provide a supportive role, behind the scenes and out of the limelight.

To reiterate, excelling in that one thing you've designated your calling will inescapably be at the expense of other areas in your life. Forget about being well-rounded. That's just a wholly unrealistic expectation, with a nice catchy ring to it. It's pure nonsense that sounds good on paper and peddled about by those that are completely clueless about what it takes to achieve actual greatness. As we touched on in the previous chapter, they may also be largely uninterested in the pursuit of elite performance or unwilling to engage in it. They're perfectly fine just dabbling at this, that, or the other, but not really excelling in any of the above. I can't tell you how many times along the way I've heard these well-rounded assailants rain on my parade with gibberish like, "I wouldn't want to be just 'book smart'...I'd rather have common sense and enjoy life experiences"—okay, have fun with that, whatever "that" means! The idea of riding shotgun to support someone else's quest for greatness could be even less appealing, especially in today's "me first" culture of instant gratification. But more on that later...

If you're still reading this far along in the book, it means you're not content with just doing the bare minimum to get by, either. Or maybe you got guilt-tripped into the being-well-rounded trap, because you didn't want to get labeled selfish or narcissistic if you focused more on your calling. But now you're secretly looking for an escape route. If that's the case, know I'm not making light of it. It's quite the opposite, in fact. I can't even pretend to have that one figured out, my friend, and I still struggle with it on a daily basis. I'd go so far as saying that the enormity of the pressure to keep those close to you feeling happy and appreciated will dictate how far you go and how fast you get there. In the end, these other competing priorities and familial obligations are what impose the heaviest time and mental constraints towards actively pursuing your dream.

Social belonging, friendships, and intimacy—these are all fundamental needs we share as human beings. It's right there with having food, shelter, and gainful employment, according to Abraham Maslow's classic "hierarchy of needs" ("A Theory of Human Motivation" in *Psychological Review,* 1943). There's no getting around that. Your family, your spouse, your kids, and your friends all want a piece of you, and vice versa. You may be able to consciously forego the fulfillment of these needs, as you plod along, but don't expect the rest of your circle to follow suit. It doesn't work that way, because you can only directly control your course of action. You can't coerce others to abide by your regimented ideology. Try as you may, but sticking to a *Lone Wolf McQuade* plan of flying solo will prove to be a real life Mission: Impossible! Take it from me; I've tried and failed miserably with that strategy. You must accept that you can't go at it alone, indefinitely. A life of solitude is no way to live, and it is incompatible with emotional stability or psychological health. It's simply not sustainable. At some point, you need to figure out how to effectively intermingle your loved ones with your mission. Like any effective leader, you have to garner buy-in from your supporting cast, which means your vision and mission statements, spoken and unspoken, must inspire them and align with their values and priorities.

How good you are at walking that tightrope and staying on course will depend on the structural integrity of the foundation you've established within your circle. That is to say, have you haphazardly thrown together a "house of cards," with virtually no wiggle room to withstand even the slightest cool breeze, or do you have a solid Rock of Gibraltar, impervious and earthquake-proof? You're only as good as your supporting cast. Not everyone gets married for the right reasons, and not all spouses or friends will acquiesce to playing second fiddle to your job or your dream. People can change over time, and having to take a backseat to your quest may get old, after a while. It's for these and an infinite number of other reasons, well beyond the scope of this little book, that you must tread carefully when navigating the minefield of life and work balance, and achieving your greatest goals. Expect both enemy fire from your detractors and friendly fire from your inner circle. By targeting all the chinks in your armor, these attacks will undoubtedly detract your attention from the quest. You'll be repeatedly asked about the merit and the sanity of your commitment with jabs like, "You don't even have a life," or, "You only care about yourself." You'll be painfully reminded of your flaws and deficiencies, and you'll be issued ultimatums about "choosing" either them or that thing you're obsessively chasing.

The pressure to conform to well-roundedness may prove too great, so you lose your nerve, and you cave. Now you're barely treading water, getting pulled in countless different directions to keep everybody else happy, and you have no idea who or what you're supposed to be anymore. You've gone from walking a tightrope to wearing a straightjacket, banging your head against a padded wall, all the while spinning your wheels. The banality of today's world may have also lost its luster for you, and your primal instincts have you yearning for something more—for legitimacy and purpose. You're not content with mediocrity, with just clocking in and out, collecting your paycheck, and heading home to finish binge-watching that great new series on Netflix. Before you know it, weeks, months, even years have whizzed by in a haze of monotonous routine and stagnant personal growth. Coasting under the radar along easy street just isn't doing it for you anymore. There's a little voice inside of you that keeps calling out to you if you listen for it. It's getting progressively louder with time, and increasingly more difficult to ignore. It's pleading for something more, much more than the status quo. Deep down, you know you were meant for so much more. Like a thoroughbred chained up in a small pen, you know you were born to run, but you're frustratingly stuck in a rut.

What we are talking about is becoming the BEST, the best you possibly can, the Michael Jordan of all the plausible versions of yourself that may come into existence. But it doesn't necessarily stop there. Beyond yourself, it could also mean daring to be the MJ of your field, someone that makes a seismic impact on the world around you, leaving it a better place than when you found it. This succinctly captures the essence of who I am to a fault. I fancy myself a "Cleaner," and I endlessly strive to become the Michael Jordan of cardiac surgery. I may very well never get there, but the thrill of the chase will always keep me in the game. It's who I am, and I refuse to deny it. In writing this book, I'm also doing my part to help others, far beyond the individual patients I care for. I've come a long way, but I'm nowhere near where I want, or need, to be.

If these sentiments also ring true for you, then you, too, may be a "Cleaner." You already are well aware that being well-rounded is overrated. The truth of the matter is that you can never be all things to all people at all times. The quest for success invariably dictates (temporary) imbalance for the greater good! Elite performance requires focused engagement and repetition. There's no way I could've simultaneously excelled in academics at an Ivy League university or top medical school, have chiseled abs, volunteered several hours a week at the homeless shelter, and started a successful small business. I had to focus! I intentionally and necessarily wasn't well-rounded. If given the choice between having world-class expertise in one area versus being a "jack-of-all-trades, master of none," I readily opt for the former. So should you. Do you really think Olympic athletes have much of "a life" when they're training all those years to win a gold medal? I think you know the answer.

The reality is that it's virtually impossible to be successful in all phases of life, simultaneously. Neil Pasricha, author of another best seller, *The Happiness Equation*, makes this point pretty clearly: "The 3 S's of Success (Social, Self, Sales) apply to all industries, professions, and aspects of life. Success is not one-dimensional. You must decide what kind of success you want….Here's the catch: It's impossible to have all three successes." I know what you're thinking. "How could something like success be so cut and dry?" Well, it all boils down to time, the time needed to accumulate the sufficient number of reps to master your craft. I tell medical students all the time, "If you can tie your shoelaces, you already have what it takes to become a heart surgeon—it's all about the reps." Practice makes perfect, and the minimum threshold for attaining mastery in any given discipline is 10,000 hours. As Malcolm Gladwell summarizes in his book *Outliers*, "Ten thousand hours is the magic number of greatness," as corroborated by several studies across various disciplines and endeavors. Roughly speaking, it takes about ten years of hard practice to hit the mark, which is, incidentally, how long it took me to complete my heart surgery training—just saying! Facts are facts, and as long as you can put in the requisite time and effort, little is beyond your reach.

The problem is there's only twenty-four hours in a day and only one of you. To rack up the 10,000 hours and the 10 years of deliberate practice necessary to attain mastery, something has to give. Who knows? Perhaps when science figures out how we can clone ourselves, we'll be able to overcome this logistical hurdle. But, until then, train your sights on your target of interest and go full court press. Visualize the win. Attack it by air, land, and sea, until you reach the key milestone you identified prior to launching this offensive. Take a (brief) breather, pat yourself on the back, and, like MJ, pinpoint the next milestone, and get right back to it! Remember, you're either all in, or it's no win. If you're not in it to win it, there's plenty of room at the kids' table!

Once you go all in, you can't look back. There will be some forks in the road that present themselves along your journey. The decision as to which route to take may feel like splitting hairs, with no clear-cut right way. In those instances, you may just have to go with your gut instinct and press on. As long as you stick to the plan and put forth every ounce of effort you can muster, it will all work out for the best. And that's precisely how my transition to the Cleveland Clinic came to pass. Rather than staying at Duke for my heart surgery training, I elected instead to throw my name in the hat for the one training spot available at the mecca of heart surgery. Duke had been great to me, and after spending eleven years there (four years of medical school and seven years of general surgery residency), it's safe to say I still bleed "Duke blue." My training at Duke had been superb, and I felt extremely well prepared to take on the world. Duke had three slots for their cardiac surgery fellowship, and I could have opted to stay for those additional three years. I love Duke, and I'm so grateful for everything I learned and experienced within the ivory towers of this storied program. But the time had come for me to explore other frontiers and to mix it up with a whole new cadre of heavy hitters and leading experts. I wanted the opportunity to get as many reps as humanly possible under the guidance and tutelage of the most prolific heart surgeons in the world.

In many regards, the Cleveland Clinic has fit the bill and continues to do so, boasting a lineup of upper echelon cardiac surgeons, having earned "Michael Jordan" status in their respective niches in the field. These technical virtuosos are frequently visited by other surgeons from the United States and abroad, hoping to watch them in action and pick up new tricks of the trade. A record three past presidents of the American Association of Thoracic Surgery (AATS), the most prestigious and exclusive of all the heart surgery professional societies, were all former chiefs at the Cleveland Clinic—Floyd Loop, Delos "Toby" Cosgrove, and Bruce Lytle. There is hardly an area of cardiac surgery or cardiology where *"the Clinic"* hasn't staked its claim as the leading center in the world or has published the largest known series with the best reported outcomes of any other center. For the past twenty plus consecutive years, it has been officially ranked the number one heart hospital in the country, according to the *U.S. News & World Report* annual rankings of the best hospitals. To put it in perspective, over 4,000 open-heart surgeries are performed at this campus on a yearly basis, more than double the number of the next busiest hospital in the nation. They don't have just the quantity. They have also the quality to back it up, consistently maintaining surgical outcomes that are second to none. From foreign dignitaries and members of the Saudi royal family to movie stars and celebrities, people from all over the world flock to Cleveland, Ohio, every year to have their heart procedures done by the very best of the best.

To meet the demands of their well-oiled machine of impeccable precision and colossal throughput, the Clinic employs a squadron of about thirty mercenary heart surgery "associates," or "super fellows," to help out in the operating room and in the postoperative care of the patients. These are fully trained heart surgeons from the United States and the four corners of the globe. We're talking the Middle East, Africa, Asia, Europe, South America, Canada, Australia—you name it. It's like a mini–United Nations battling out in the trenches of the Heart and Vascular Institute of the Cleveland Clinic. Many are looking to home in on a specific subspecialty of cardiac surgery or are wanting to jump-start their careers back in their native countries. Some are several years out from their heart surgery training and are therefore seasoned vets in this specialty. Thrown into the mix was the lowly "board resident." That was me, the one individual selected every year to "learn" heart surgery essentially from scratch, having only completed training in general surgery.

I guess they figured taking the extra time to teach one person the fine art of heart surgery wouldn't appreciably slow down the machine. Indeed, the learning curve is mind-blowingly steep, and the stakes don't get any higher. As a fully trained general surgeon, I felt extremely comfortable and technically competent navigating my way through the organs of the abdomen and through the blood vessels in the neck and the extremities. Heck, I just survived Duke Surgery! But as I found out pretty quickly, heart surgery is a whole other ball game, and I was starting back at the bottom of the totem pole. The heart is a moving target, not a stationary organ, like the liver, the spleen, or the brain. Makes you wonder why the saying, "It's not *brain* surgery," came to pass—I propose we change it to, "It's not *heart* surgery," instead! Of course, I may be biased, but hear me out, as I plead my case. Every single step of a cardiac operation, from beginning to end, is fraught with life-threatening danger. Even the slightest misstep can be fatal for the patient (and fatal for your career prospects). Just opening the chest itself, the first step of any cardiac surgery, can result in fatal exsanguination, if you misjudge the anatomic location of the heart and lacerate it with your sternal saw. There's danger lurking at every turn.

Heart surgeons must face the same somber reality every time they leave home for "work." A bad day at the office means someone passes away and that person's blood is on your hands. You either thrive on that level of accountability and stress, or you crumble under the weight of its mounting pressure. It's not for everyone, and it sure as hell isn't for anyone not willing to go all in!

The great ones stay on an even keel, never losing their cool, and always in control of whatever mishap presents itself. They lead by example, and if anything goes awry, they take responsibility for it. By not pointing fingers, they avoid the ABCDs of failure (Accuse, Blame, Criticize, and Defer). One of the most heavily scrutinized surgical procedures in the United States is coronary artery bypass grafting (CABG) for heart-artery blockages. Perfection is the expectation. The procedure entails creating alternate routes of blood traffic, by using segments of veins or arteries (harvested from the legs, arms, or ribcage) and sewing them directly to the coronary artery downstream from the point where the blockages are located. The manual dexterity necessary to suture bypass grafts onto one-to-two-millimeter-in-diameter coronary arteries is daunting. The needles used are the size of an eyelash attached to a suture that's comparable to a hair strand in size and tensile strength. The coronary artery wall of diseased vessels is typically very friable and as thin as tissue paper. Being able to reliably tie these sutures down without breaking them, but tightly enough so the suture line doesn't leak like a sieve, is a massive undertaking to master, requiring thousands upon thousands of reps.

We haven't even touched on the fact that there's quite the time crunch in heart surgery, so you don't have all day to pull off these procedural wonders. The longer you have the heart stopped to fix or replace whatever's necessary, the greater the risk for bleeding, for damage to other organs, and for injury to the heart itself. How's that for pressure? You can buy some time, up to a couple of hours, by cooling the body down and administering a variety of sophisticated "cardioplegic" fluids to keep the heart copacetic while it's arrested. But that said, time is of the essence, and you're ideally getting the job done as expeditiously as humanly possible. You must sew like the wind, and there can be no wasted moves. Don't forget to make sure everything is flawlessly sewn, because if any of your suture lines leak later, your patient will bleed to death in the ICU. To me, the time constraints and the necessity for such economy of motion set heart surgery apart from any other kind of surgery, by leaps and bounds. That's where I'll rest my case on the "it's not heart surgery" instead of "it's not brain surgery" argument. Much love and no disrespect intended to my talented brainiac neurosurgeons out there!

There is no margin for error in heart surgery. At the Clinic, you were always one mistake away from being benched, much like an NFL quarterback jockeying for the starting position who throws an interception in a preseason game. He'll likely be riding the pine until further notice, if he's lucky enough to even earn a spot on the team roster. Likewise, there was always a fully trained super fellow warming up in the bullpen, ready to assume my place at the OR table, if I whiffed. As long as you kept bringing the heat and throwing strikes, you were allowed to stay in the game. When given an opportunity to sew, you had to make it count. You had to shine, because if you didn't, your next shot could be a ways away. If I wasn't physically in the operating room or taking care of patients on the wards, I practiced my suturing morning, noon, and night, on all manner of household props, including wet tissue paper set in a shoebox. As if that wasn't enough, I also found time to work on a number of clinical research projects and manuscripts with a few of the faculty. This led to approximately ten publications in cardiac-surgery journals during my stint in Cleveland. Heart surgery became my life. I went all in!

To put it mildly, I sold my soul to this endeavor and to the Clinic. As my skills steadily improved, my confidence soared, and I gained increasing trust from the faculty. I was promoted to "chief resident" during the beginning of my second year, earlier than the majority of the board residents had in the past. Like a kid feasting in a candy store, I was operating like a fiend on an almost daily basis, living and working in the Zone. People often asked me if I minded the cold and gloomy weather of the "'Mistake on the Lake.'" Quite honestly, I grew very fond of Cleveland and didn't get bothered by the inclement weather. Part of it may have to do with the fact that I didn't see the light of day for the three years I spent there—I could never get enough of the bright lights of the operating room, doing what I loved and learning from the best!

Because of the sheer volume and extensive breadth of

complexity of patients we were seeing, the training I received was just out of this world. Despite all the sleepless nights, grueling hours, and unimaginable stress, I couldn't imagine doing anything else, and I felt tremendously thankful for this learning opportunity. You can't help getting comfortable with handling the worst-case scenario or with the rarest of the rare disasters, because you were repeatedly exposed to them on a regular basis. It was Disney World for heart surgeons, except that its doors never closed. Our norm would, in most other places, be everyone else's nightmare, but we welcomed the misery with open arms—bring it! There's something to be said for that added level of preparation. It was constant repetition that desensitized you to chaos and that made you ready to rock at the drop of a dime. During my final weeks, I posed for this picture in front of the main entrance to the operating rooms, where a big sign on the wall read, "Through These Portals Pass the World's Greatest Cardiothoracic and Vascular Surgical Teams" (please disregard the nicely trimmed goatee I was sporting, as this was all the rage at the time; no, seriously, I swear it was). In it, I was donning the standard issued "whites" worn by the surgeons at the Clinic. Rather than typical surgical scrubs which were totally played out, we preferred the vintage white uniform, reminiscent of a very highly trained milkman!

But in as much as the OR was my happy place and safe haven, where I thrived and everything made sense, my personal life outside of the OR was in a shambles. Like a fish out of water, I couldn't adjust well to the mundanities of civilian life, such as taking out the trash, keeping things tidy, hearing about how "hard" someone else's day was—ugh, get me back to the OR, pronto! Technically speaking, while I was married

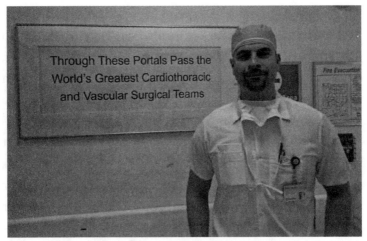

Entrance to operating rooms during my final weeks of heart-surgery training at the Cleveland Clinic, 2012.

at the time, it was a union that existed purely on paper and was doomed from the beginning—my true bride and first love was heart surgery, as if you already didn't know! The truth is I didn't get married for the right reasons, and I had failed to think my decision through all the way. I approached it like just another checkbox on my "to-do list." Marriage seemed more like something I was supposed to do at that stage of my career. It was just another rite of passage. Most of my colleagues were married with kids, and I was long overdue for the same, or so I thought. This cringe-worthy logic made perfect sense at the time, and that goes to show how you how profoundly brain-washed I had become. It would be a few years before I finally realized what holy matrimony was really all about, when I met the true love of my life, Courtney, and remarried three years ago. I learned that marriage is a sacred institution that requires giving up part of yourself, your identity, for the sake and sanctity of this new union with this special person with whom you've committed to spend the rest of your life.

Back in my Cleveland days, however, I wasn't willing to give an inch. They say absence makes the heart grow fonder, but when there's indefinite absence that's not only physical in nature, then there's no room for improvement or anything to look forward to. I was an absentee husband, literally and figuratively. For someone so attuned to critical illness and adept at saving lives, I was a rank amateur at recognizing my own marriage was on life support from the moment we exchanged our vows. It barely lasted a couple of years, but it was really over before it started. I had no business getting married or dragging anyone along on this crazy ride. The depth of my marital ineptitude was primarily driven by my inability to equitably balance the wants and needs of another person into the single-minded madness that had taken over my life at that time. I hadn't figured that part out yet. The price I personally paid for going all in was losing myself completely in the process. That's the dark side of going all in, because it's hard to shut the switch off, when you're always in attack mode. My entire identity was wrapped up in being a heart surgeon. I had no clue who Brian Lima even was anymore. I especially couldn't recognize that pudgy dude in the mirror looking back at me who clearly had let himself go of late. I suddenly found myself in the throes of a full blown identity crisis!

Newly divorced, out of shape, and burned out, I arrived at yet another major crossroads. The cumulative effects of going all in, all those years, had taken their toll. My training was finally complete, and I couldn't wait to leave the nest and to spread my wings. It felt so surreal! I was a full-fledged cardiothoracic surgeon, with special training in heart transplant and mechanical circulatory support (MCS)—using artificial heart technology to support those with advanced or irreversible heart failure. Gone were the days of scraping by, miserably living paycheck to paycheck, and I breathed a huge sigh of relief. Now I had to figure out where to hang out my shingle and make my official "adulting" debut as a new member of the grownup workforce. Would I be taking my talents to the academic stage and leave my indelible mark on heart surgery, like so many of the legendary greats that mentored and trained me? Or would I eschew notoriety, join a nice private practice, and ride off into the sunset of academic obscurity, leaving that stuffy world behind? My pedigree, track record, and CV all pointed towards academia. I was bred to be a triple threat, to push the envelope of innovation in the field of cardiac surgery and to help train the next generation of heart surgeons. All signs resoundingly pointed to that eventuality, but the fire that had burned so bright for so long in my belly had been unceremoniously extinguished in the wake of my failed marriage and newfound disenchantment with my life as a whole outside of the OR. The problem was I had my fill of the hamster wheel and wasn't too keen on further engaging in the "publish or perish," operate-until-you-drop, painful climb up the academic ladder. After having not come up for air in nearly two decades, I needed to regroup. To guide my next move, I would base my decision on what was best for "Brian Lima." The person, not "Brian Lima" the heart surgeon. This was an unprecedented departure from my modus operandi and ushered in a wave of much-needed change in my life going forward.

Sure, I made my rounds, interviewing at various prestigious places, the usual suspects, with all that swagger, pomp, and circumstance I had come to expect as business as usual. What many of these blowhards didn't know was that I was just going through the motions. It didn't help matters that there was virtually no wining and dining, or rolling out of the red carpet—I could barely get my trip expenses or hotel stay reimbursed. The prestige of the name alone was supposed to sell itself, so why bother making you feel wanted or even welcome? Perks? You get to have "*Fancy* University Medical Center" stationary, with your name on it. I should be so lucky! A year or two prior, I would have killed for a faculty position at any number of places like this, but things had changed. Believe me: I felt more than qualified and deserving of these lofty positions, but my priorities had shifted. I needed to think about what was best for me and not just what was best for my career. Some healing time was in order, and that's what I set my sights on finding.

Success had become almost like an addiction that consumed me, a common phenomenon among many overachievers, who likewise feel compelled to step away, to refocus, and to recharge their engines. The good news, as Grover points out in *Relentless*, is that after this therapeutic sabbatical, Cleaners "usually return with a renewed appetite for even more." That's precisely what happened to me. I joined CTVS (Cardiothoracic & Vascular Surgeons), a private practice group in Austin, Texas, and really had the time of my life. It felt like I was part of a family, a fraternal order of the best partners and colleagues you could ever possibly ask for, in one of the hippest and trendiest cities in the country. Over the course of about two years, I got back into good physical shape and rediscovered who I was. Not only did I become human again; I also came into my own as a surgeon and was loving every minute, both inside the OR and outside of it.

Life as a heart surgeon in Austin was a far cry from the

frenzied pace I had grown accustomed to for the better part of my adult life. It's not to say that CTVS didn't operate a lot or take great care of its patients. The volume of work and number of patients was more manageable, however, lending itself to work-life balance. For the first time in a very long time, I had more free time on my hands than I knew what to do with, and I tried to make the most of it. The warm weather and the beautiful Town Lake afforded a host of outdoor activities that I enjoyed. I traveled, visited family, and took full advantage of the smorgasbord of offerings the "live music capital of the United States" had on the menu! The party scene was alive and well, and no matter what day of the week it was, there was never any shortage of live performances or other fun events to attend.

A sign of the times not unique to Austin, I'm sure, was just how over-the-top the party scene had become. I was shocked to learn that "Sunday Funday" was an actual thing! The bars and clubs were packed, and everyone was partying it up on Sundays like it was 1999. Day of rest? Who are you kidding? I remember thinking, "What fresh hell is this? Does anybody in this town work for a living?" Having never gotten completely over the whole "Thursday is the new Friday" partygoer movement that began when I was in college, I was utterly flabbergasted that debauchery could sink to such depths. I could barely stomach one late night out a week, much less four! How fitting that the party anthem "Turn Down for What" by Lil John was released around this time to provide the perfect theme music for all of these shenanigans. I've got to hand it to you, millennials, you really know how to have fun! By comparison, I'm likely the tamest and lamest "party animal" you'll ever lay eyes on, who rarely stays up past my bedtime, unless

I'm operating on someone's heart.

It took a while for me to acclimate to this laid-back lifestyle and to part with my curmudgeon tendencies. Things were really coming together nicely, and I could feel myself becoming whole again. To top it all off, Austin is the city where I eventually met and fell in love with my future wife, Courtney! When you put it all together, it's no wonder that, throughout CTVS's fifty-year history, all the surgeons that joined the group stayed for their entire surgical careers, with rare exception. It's hard to envision a more idyllic setting to live, work, and play. The utopian ambiance was rubbing off on me, and there were times when I, too, could see myself spending the rest of my life in Austin. I came very close to doing so, and, for a second there, I even entertained the idea of wearing cowboy boots in the OR, like many of my homegrown Texan partners.

But as much as I tried to convince myself that this was the "happily ever after" ending I deserved, I knew there was still some unfinished business I needed to tend to—my inner MJ voice had resurfaced and began whispering sweet nothings into my ear. The Cleaner was coaxing me back onto the battlefield to fulfill my true destiny, and it wasn't taking "no" for answer. I was now fully recharged, reinvigorated, and repurposed to resume my quest for greatness. My ambition was like a sleeping giant reawakened from its hibernating state—bigger, bolder, and better equipped to meet the demands of the next leg on my arduous journey. This time around, I had a much firmer grasp of who I was, what I wanted to become, and how I wanted to get there!

The first stop on my comeback campaign would be Baylor University Medical Center (BUMC) in Dallas, Texas. "Everything is bigger in Texas," so it's saying a lot when you consider that BUMC is the largest hospital in the entire Dallas-Fort Worth Metroplex, which, oh, by the way, encompasses about 7 million people. A relative unknown on the cardiac surgery scene, BUMC was an institution with a chip on its shoulder, looking to blaze new trails and make waves in the heart-surgery world. To that end, they elected to ramp up their heart-transplant program by recruiting a highly touted team of surgeons from the Cleveland Clinic. In record time, the program grew by leaps and bounds, as this special ops crew stormed the castle, predictably taking no prisoners and taking the heart failure world by storm. When the opportunity to stage this hostile takeover of Dallas was initially floated, I was offered the right of first refusal, but I had already committed to my deal in Austin. We were all buddies, like-minded individuals that went way back, having slogged it out together in the heart-surgery trenches for years. So we kept in touch, as our mutually exclusive missions took on lives of their own.

Within months of starting my Austin gig, my old friends began periodically checking in to see if I had a change of heart. Almost overnight, BUMC had suddenly become a true force to be reckoned with as one of the busiest heart-transplant centers in the country. My old friends were drowning and in desperate need of reinforcements. Before long, I became progressively receptive to their advances for a number of reasons. It was do-or-die time for me, and I had to make my move. The longer I stayed out of academia, the more challenging it would be to reach my full potential. I was ready to reenter the fray, and I fortuitously found my road to redemption. This was a golden opportunity that fell in my lap, and I couldn't squander it. As one of the primary heart-transplant surgeons in one of the nation's highest-volume programs, I would be uniquely positioned to help push the envelope in heart-transplant science. By overseeing the research efforts in the BUMC heart failure space, I would be serving as principal investigator for clinical trials involving the latest advances in mechanical heart-pump technology. I would also be serving as the Surgical Director of Mechanical Circulatory Support, tasked with helping build and grow a premiere surgical heart failure program. This package deal was a no-brainer, so I signed on the dotted line and headed north, leaving Austin in my rearview mirror. Just as Michael Corleone said in *The Godfather Part III,* "Just when I thought I was out, they pull me back in!"

This chapter's long enough already, so I won't bore you with what happened next! It'll be covered in the upcoming chapters, but let's just say it all worked out for the best. It's time now for our parting shots, as we close out what is deservedly the longest chapter in the book. When you go all in, it means you're in it to win it. You're in it for the long haul, and you're willing to accept the consequences that come along with your steadfast efforts! There's a hefty price to be paid for chasing your dreams that's nonnegotiable. It could mean sacrificing other parts of your life, being disproportionately focused on your calling and far from well-rounded. You can lose yourself in the process, as I did, and struggle to find your way back. If you're really living *the Heart Way,* it means you're going all in to be the best possible version of yourself that you can in the service of your calling. No dream is too big, but nothing comes easy. Don't settle for anything less than your best because you're better than that, and your calling deserves your best. If it's really your calling, much of this may come naturally—it won't feel like "work" per se.

Don't misconstrue "a calling" for something that has to be

earth shattering, that has to garner lots of dollar signs, or that has to attract millions of followers on social media. On the contrary, the desire for glitz and glamour or fame and fortune should never be your primary driver. A lot of that has to do with staying grounded, balanced, and attentive to the welfare of those close to you. Don't make the same mistake I made, and don't think you can carry the load yourself. Relationships are key, and both your humanity and sanity depend on them. Having people in your corner through the highs and the lows, through victories and defeats, is priceless! Don't let them fall by the wayside. What good is it to fulfill your dream if you don't have anyone to share it with? Do the right thing, and get after it!

"If not YOU, then WHO?
If not NOW, then WHEN?
No more questions.
GET AFTER IT!"
–BRIAN LIMA

CHAPTER 9

NOT FOR THE FAINT OF *HEART*: HAVE NO FEAR

"Big time players make big time plays in big time games."
—SANTANA MOSS

"Let me assert my firm belief that the only thing we have to fear is...fear itself—nameless, unreasoning, unjustified terror which paralyzes needed efforts to convert retreat into advance."—FRANKLIN D. ROOSEVELT

With all due respect to former President FDR, there may be a few instances when retreating in fear is an absolute must, if you value your life. Say, for instance, you're getting charged by a wild rhino while on a safari expedition in South Africa. Fresh off a successful big-game hunt, you've unknowingly instigated a clash with Mother Nature, and she's looking to even the score. As you're alone and unarmed, only dimwitted bravery, or just plain old "beer muscles," would compel you to play chicken with this hooved bulldozer. Talk about carnage—guess who winds up on the losing end of that collision? Standing your ground may be the appropriate tactic with many other animal encounters, such as those with bears or wolves, because running away may only incite the chase. But you don't have to be Jane Goodall or some other expert zoologist to know that a charging rhino is one glaring exception to that rule. The excess safari booze may have dulled your senses, but, luckily for you, your adrenaline-induced "fight-or-flight response" will still have you instinctively barreling towards the nearest tree to climb—faster than a gazelle on PEDs (performance enhancing drugs)! Be thankful that evolution has graciously hardwired this survival instinct into our sympathetic nervous system, an autonomic cascade of neurohormonal events triggered solely by "fear." Think of it as nature's "panic button." Without it, no member of the animal kingdom could ever successfully navigate the savagery of the unforgiving wild.

This defense mechanism sure comes in handy when you're life is in danger, but such events are few and far between in today's modern world, right? At least not within the humdrum confines of the concrete jungles the vast majority of us call home? Unlike the prehistoric days of our ancient ancestors, when evading saber-toothed tigers and other occupational hazards were part and parcel of their hunter-gatherer lifestyle, it's not every day we're faced with the imminent threat posed by other species. Short of the occasional household pet "gone wild" or overzealous zookeeper, such events have become as infrequent and random as being struck by lightning. That being said, you would think this evolutionary adaptation is largely vestigial within our civilized existence, suffering the same fate as our appendix, our wisdom teeth, and our tailbone—an atrophied relic we carry around like a souvenir, a throwback to harsher times many millennia ago. I wish that were the case. For a variety of reasons, the opposite has occurred. Even though it's the "safest" time in human history, we're, paradoxically, more scared than ever, as Neil Strauss recounts in his 2016 *Rolling Stone* article entitled "We're Living in the Age of Fear." It seems our panic buttons are stuck in the "on" position.

That may sound like a tough pill to swallow. But it makes complete sense, when you think about how hectic modern-day life has become. As humans, we've ascended to the top of the food chain, becoming the apex predator and the master of all species on Earth. It's good to be king, but no reign lasts forever. Just ask T-Rex and his dinosaur compadres. Before abdicating the throne, they ran the show for over 200 *million* years, with no signs of letting up. Had Mother Nature not stepped in, we might very well have missed our turn at bat. Considering modern humans have only been around for a paltry 200 *thousand* years, the dinosaurs have set the bar pretty high with their impressive run. So we better get our act together if we have any hope of eclipsing that mark. But it's regrettably not looking very promising, if you ask me, because, unlike the dinosaurs, we've turned on ourselves. The greatest existential threats we face come courtesy of our own species. In the absence of any plausible threats to our species' dominance, we've somehow become our own worst enemy! Can't we all just get along?

If today's world has become a scary place, it's because WE have made it that way! We are constantly devising new, sick, and twisted ways to hurt ourselves and one another. Just take a gander at all the headlines, and you'll get the idea—recurrent and recycled variations of the same scary stuff over and over again, an onslaught of BREAKING NEWS streaming 24/7 on network news stations, flooding the Internet, or pinging alerts on our smartphones: *another* school shooting, sex trafficking, global warming, carjacking, foreign trade wars, the federal deficit, the EBOLA virus, the opioid epidemic, stock market crash, government shutdowns, identity theft, cyberbullying, cyberwarfare, religious extremists, weapons of mass destruction, terrorists, bioterrorism, and suicide bombers. Is it just me? Or did you also have to pause midway and stave off a full blown panic attack? Ladies and gentlemen, welcome to "the most fearmongering time in human history," as author Barry Glassner describes in his book *The Culture of Fear*.

The media would have you thinking that the sky is falling. The truth of the matter is that it's never been safer to be human than it is today, with unprecedented lows in crime rates, in famine, in disease, and in war, relative to any other point in our short history on this planet. According to Glassner, "Most Americans are living in the safest place at the safest time in human history." But for the power brokers and media giants, that hardly qualifies as a newsworthy headline—fear sells, and there are billions to be made at our expense. To boost their ratings and to continue raking in the dough, they perpetuate our fears by sensationalizing the macabre, by catastrophizing, and by overreporting the evils that men do. Playing to our morbid curiosity, they reel us in with nonstop train wrecks and car crashes, and we can't help gawking like rubbernecking motorists slowing down to check out the wreckage on the side of the road. Striking fear in the hearts of the masses is also an ingenious tactic employed by those with politically motivated agendas seeking to sway our votes in upcoming elections.

Nothing stirs a crowd more than manipulative propaganda, scapegoating, fearmongering and other mind games—the sine qua non of today's predominantly partisan political landscape.

Speaking of politics, you had better be exquisitely careful about what you say and how you say it. Speak freely? Or "off the record?" Guess again. Forget about context or frame of reference and how your words *should* be interpreted. You need to think twice about speaking your mind, because anything you say can and will be used against you in the court of public opinion. The omnipresent PC police will instantly pounce on any statement they perceive as "offensive" or "insensitive,'" so a word to the wise—mind your p's and q's at all times. Such is the climate of our "callout culture" and "gotcha journalism," where even the slightest, totally inadvertent verbal misstep can have disastrous consequences—you can go from a virtual unknown to public enemy number one, with just a single, misworded tweet, sound bite, or misrepresented quotation taken "out of context."

This inflated sense of danger in the world keeps us in a perpetually hypervigilant state of consternation. Our trigger-happy fight-or-flight response is set on overdrive. Everything is a potential threat in this perfect storm of widespread paranoia and fear, so we never ever carelessly throw caution to the wind. It's all about "just in case" or "you never know"—precaution and preoccupation with the falling sky. There are no molehills left—only mountains! We live in gated communities, lock our doors at night, and activate our home-security alarm systems, complete with surveillance cameras, motion-sensor floodlights, video doorbells, and even "panic rooms"—you know, *just in case* your home intruders manage to MacGyver their way inside. No cause for concern there, because you're armed to the teeth with a military grade arsenal of assault weapons to choose from, for *self-defense*—because you never know.

We have GPS tracking devices for our cars, kids, and pets, *just in case* any of them are lost, stolen, or abducted. The scourge of gun violence and school shootings has further intensified our collective level of dread and trepidation, regardless of where you stand on the gun-control debate. Most schools now regularly conduct "active shooter drills," and many have incorporated armed guards and metal detectors, *just in case.* These and other real-world issues have spawned the culture of "safetyism" described in *The Coddling of the American Mind* as "the cult of safety—an obsession with eliminating threats (both real and imagined)...that deprives young people of the experiences that their antifragile minds need, thereby making them more fragile, anxious, and prone to seeing themselves as victims."

Professionally speaking, I can attest to how the preponderance of nonsensical fear has negatively impacted the prognosis of the over 100,000 people on the transplant waiting list. According to the latest organ donation statistics (www.organ-donor.gov/statistics-stories/statistics.html), only 58 percent of U.S. adults are signed up to be organ donors, further compounding the donor-organ shortage. As a result, twenty people die every day waiting for a transplant that never comes, because many people are fearful about committing themselves to become organ donors. They're afraid that doing so would somehow hasten their own demise, should they ever become critically ill. The premise for this preposterous urban legend is that health care workers, upon learning of an individual's organ-donor status, "wouldn't try as hard" to save that patient, settling instead for the consolation prize of organ donation.

I truly hope you don't believe that and can appreciate how utterly absurd and unfounded this myth is—it can't possibly be any further from the truth. Morally and ethically, this runs counter to every fabric of our being as physicians and our Hippocratic Oath. It would never happen, and, if anything, we're often so reluctant to admit defeat that we tend to prolong "end-of-life care" objectively beyond the point of medical futility. So, please, if you haven't done so already, kindly register to become an organ donor at your earliest convenience. Don't allow unreasonable fear to needlessly claim the lives of eight other people who would benefit from your donation, should you suffer an untimely death. I'll get off my soapbox now, kind of...

Technology was intended to make our lives easier, but, if anything, it's made us infinitely more stressed, always on the clock, and completely reliant on digital transactions. Your identity, your livelihood, and your finances are now open game and susceptible to attack by computer-savvy criminals. You can never be too safe these days, because the consequences of letting your guard done can be very grave. That fact has been painfully hammered into us. Every single one of our email accounts, apps, handheld devices, and bank accounts is password-protected to shield our identities and our finances from cyberattacks. The threat of being hacked is ever-present, with constantly evolving virulence, like that of drug-resistant bacteria. For those of us that work in health care, we're held legally accountable for the privacy and the security of our patients' protected health information. Failure to comply with any of the federal regulations spelled out in the Health Insurance Portability and Accountability Act (HIPAA) can lead to hefty fines or actual jail time. Yikes! As a result, our login passwords to access the electronic health record (EHR) are forcibly reset about as often as you change your bedsheets—add that to an exponentially growing collection of passwords few of us can barely manage, if at all. I miss paper charts! I miss paper in general!

We live in a giant pressure cooker, on constant alert and with an overactive fear response. It can be exhausting to live this way, and, more often than not, I find myself longing for simpler times. You know things are bad when the stress of the world has you seriously contemplating roughing it in the wilderness and fending for yourself. It may not exactly be hitting rock bottom, but, for a city slicker like me, fantasizing about the wonders of survivalism is pretty darn close. It's not surprising that nearly one-third of U.S. adults experience a serious anxiety disorder at some point during their lives, according to the National Institute of Mental Health (www.nimh.nih.gov), with similar prevalence noted among adolescents (aged thirteen to eighteen). What's more, over 34 million Americans report having a phobia, and they collectively dole out over $7 billion every year for therapies aimed at resolving their fear (www.couponbox.com/press/fighting-fear-the-7-billion-dollar-price-tag/).

Fear is big business, with projected growth that will likely be off the charts at the rate we're going. It's muscled its way into the natural order of things, at both the individual level and society as a whole. According to Hendrie Weisinger and J. P. Pawliw-Fry, authors of the book *Performing Under Pressure,* with so many of us afflicted with anxiety, we may be prone to "an exaggerated perception of threat" which triggers "fear that is so strong it dominates logical thinking, replacing it with overwhelming feelings of anxiety and fear, reminiscent of the primal but realistic panic our ancestors experienced in their face-to-face encounters with predators."

Sound familiar? It does to me. I freely admit that many of my fears are illogical and primally driven, such as my fear of clowns, sharks, and FAILURE—yes, failure! Known as "aty-chiphobia," fear of failure has been a lifelong struggle of mine. Apparently, I'm not alone. Fear of personal failure was the most commonly reported phobia in the survey mentioned above. That brings us to the meat of this chapter. But before diving in here, there are a few disclaimers that bear mentioning. First off, if you've come to this chapter looking for insights and practical advice related to conquering your fear of failure, you've come to the right place. Conversely, if sharks scare the bejesus out of you, as they do me, you're definitely barking up the wrong tree. I'm fresh out of answers and a self-proclaimed *total wuss* when it comes to swimming in the deep blue sea. My irrational fear of sharks, or galeophobia, as it is officially termed, and all aquatic wildlife, for that matter, can be traced back to the movie *Jaws*, and I've been plagued with it ever since. You couldn't pay me enough to hop into one of those shark cages to "observe" them in their natural environment. Scratch that—forget money; you'd have to fully anesthetize me to play along. I don't care if the cage was made out of Adamantium and if Aqua Man himself was there to chaperone the encounter, the closest I'm ever getting to these oceanic monsters is *Shark Week* on the Discovery Channel!

While we're at it, we might as well throw in claustrophobia, agarophobia, and the umpteen other "phobias" in the mix. Just like galeophobia, I've got nothing for you. But don't fret, because there's only one kind of fear that's relevant to our discussion. It isn't the fear of getting eaten alive or plummeting

to your death from high altitudes that sabotages choke art-
ists in the big game or that prevents casual observers from
ever becoming relevant movers and shakers. We're going all
in on ridding the fear factor holding you and countless others
back from reaching your full potential—your fear of failure.
But, first, let's take a selfie!—kidding, but I had you there for
a second, didn't I? Maybe? Okay, but, seriously, let's frame the
discussion around another—yes, you guessed it—sports analogy. And this one's a doozy—the last-second heroics of the
game-winning shot and who's stepping up to take it!

As we delve deep into the bowels of fear and failure, I want
you to think about the dialogue you have with yourself whenever major challenges or opportunities present themselves.
Does your heart rate go way up and your mind start racing as
you whip yourself up into a frenzy? Are you so risk-averse and
quick to talk yourself out of "going for it" because you keep
perseverating on everything that could go wrong? "What if I
miss? What if I mess up or choke?" What a load of baloney!
Unshackling yourself from this negative self-talk and building
your self-confidence could be the major breakthrough you've
been waiting for, so buckle up and enjoy the ride! Here goes
nothing…

Permit me first to set the stage, by providing a little background. You probably already know that every great team has
one—the "big time" player that all the other players and fans
look to when the game is on the line and they need a miracle.
They've been here before, and they've witnessed their Cleaner
work his magic, like "Air" Jordan in the Zone, clutch performance after clutch performance. You heard all about these
types of individuals in the last chapter. In these pressure situations, they just stay as cool as a cucumber, unfazed by all the

drama. It's no secret who's getting the ball and taking the final shot! All the spectators in the stands, the people watching on TV from home, the opposing team members, and even the sports announcers know it's all coming down to whether the Cleaner hits the shot or not! You'll often here the commentator just come out and say it on the broadcast, "In these situations, 'so and so' always wants the ball in his hands!"

To add to the drama, the game's already extended into overtime, and my wife's becoming visibly panic-stricken. The new episode of *The Bachelor* started twenty minutes ago, and she can't bear the thought of inadvertently learning the outcome of the rose ceremony, while scrolling through her newsfeed. "It'll be okay, honey. There's only three minutes left in overtime" I calmly explain, hoping to allay her fears. "You said that twenty minutes ago," she screeches back, seeing right through the B.S. of the so-called "game clock." Finally, six time-outs, five commercial breaks, and about thirty minutes later, the Cleaner gets the ball and lets it fly—swoosh! Nothing but net, and the crowd goes wild! Another one for the record books and another night sleeping in the guestroom of the Lima doghouse for yours truly!

Joking aside, through sports, we catch a good glimpse of how pressure situations can bring out the best and the worst in us, depending on how well-adapted we are to handling stressful circumstances. Some players step up and fearlessly accept the challenge, as just another day at the office, business as usual. They're meant for that moment, built to meet that challenge, and willing to accept whatever happens. Others, however, are all too happy to pass the ball to the Cleaner, not wanting to have the outcome fall on their shoulders or to face the ridicule and judgement of the masses if they fall short.

They're afraid of failure and tap out. The pressure psyched them out and activated their panic buttons. That's fear in a nutshell, a true microcosm of choking under pressure. The truth is that the closer we are to being "like Mike"—fearless and confident—the better we fare in all pressure situations, on and off the court, in all facets of life.

Let's be clear; overcoming fear is a monumental task. Just like conquering any other phobia, it will require meeting your fear head-on, again and again, until you're desensitized to its paralyzing influence. If I were dead set on ridding my fear of sharks, which, for the record, I'm not, but, hypothetically speaking, if I actually was, then I would force myself to repeatedly dive into shark cages. Over time, and with each successive dive, I'd become increasingly comfortable around these cute little fishies. Hopefully, I wouldn't get maimed in the process.

There's no way around it. Life is a contact sport, and there's no way you can learn something or become expert at it, without taking your licks. It's dangerous and scary, but the more you do it, the less you are scared of it. You understand that there's risk involved. You're not cavalier about it, but you don't fear it. Call it a "healthy respect" for the magnitude of the task at hand. But you don't let fear hold you back, because you're afraid of failure. You step up to the plate, and you take the shot.

To be that big-time player, you can never allow the moment to be bigger than you are—no moment is too big or too small. They're just moments. You just need to do you, in the Zone, at that moment, and forget that anything or anyone else exists. That's me when I'm doing open-heart surgery. And that's exactly how Christian Laetner executed one of the greatest plays in the history of sports. Let me explain. I wasn't always a diehard Duke basketball fan, and Duke wasn't always the perennial juggernaut of college basketball that everyone loves to hate. That all came to pass in 1992, when "Coach K" still went by Coach Mike Krzyzewski and when the Blue Devils were just an upstart team, only one year removed from their first NCAA National Championship. Down 102-103 with 2.1 seconds left against Kentucky in the Eastern Regional Final, Coach K called a time-out. Even though I was not yet a huge college basketball fan, the game happened to be televised, and I was slightly intrigued to see its conclusion. Little did I know that I was witnessing history, a game that many would later regard as one of the greatest ever played in the NCAA tournament. Christian Laetner, Duke's 6'11" star forward, had played a picture-perfect game, scoring thirty-one points and not missing a single shot! That was impressive, to say the least, but I still had my doubts. During the time-out, I vividly recall thinking, "No way Duke pulls this one out!" Sure enough, Laetner catches the inbound pass, fakes out a defender, and gets off a clean shot that hits nothing but net, with time running out! I flew off the sofa screaming, because I just saw the impossible happen. Known simply as "The Shot," Laetner's epic buzzer beater is among the greatest moments in all of sports annals, and Duke went on to win the NCAA National Championship that year, then three more times (2001, 2010, and 2015).

Now that's what you call a clutch performance! So what do big-time players have that other nominal players lack? They've mastered pressure. Said another way, they don't acknowledge pressure; it doesn't register as a blip on their radar. No matter the situation—practice, regular-season game, championship—it's just business as usual, and they conduct themselves the same way every time. With a fight-or-flight response that's on permanent vacation, they never panic or play it safe. Do you think Laetner was worried about the ramifications of missing that legendary shot? No; it was automatic, just another shot, like the thousands he took in practice every week. You see, choking happens when we allow the pressure of the situation to make us overthink what we're doing instead of just trusting our instincts and our abilities, like riding a bike. We put extra pressure on ourselves by assigning greater importance to the moment at hand, and we freeze up, hesitate, and perform well below our capabilities. In her book *Choke*, Sian Beilock referred to this cognitive distortion as "paralysis by analysis." For an activity that normally requires no conscious thought, we start nervously focusing on details that throw us off our game. By trying harder than usual, we end up screwing it up, as Beilock describes:

> "When people are concerned about themselves and their performance, they tend to try to control their movements in order to ensure an optimal outcome; but if you're executing a skill you have done a thousand times in the past, the overattention that ensues when you are trying to perform at your best is exactly what makes you fall flat on your face."

As a heart surgeon, I encounter the threat of these cognitive distortions on a daily basis. The typical example that I and many of my surgical colleagues run into a lot is that of the "VIP patient." For whatever reason, whether it's wealth, power, fame, or all three, this individual is a big deal and commands "special treatment." The team is noticeably uptight, with body language screaming, "We'd better not screw this one up." I always chuckle to myself in these scenarios, because, as with the Cleaner taking the final shot, I do heart surgery the same way every time. I always pull out all the stops—all in, every patient, every day. Regardless of whether you're the president of the United States, the billionaire CEO of a Fortune 500 company, or some homeless guy living in a shelter, you're getting the same meticulous attention to detail during your heart procedure that I give every single one of my patients. That's the beautiful thing about medicine—human physiology is blind to race, color, creed, or socioeconomic status. There is no "VIP tray of surgical instruments" that I request specifically for this patient or that patient. There is no deviation from the operative plan or sequence of steps. It's when you start to get cute, to improvise, or to overthink what you're doing, that you flub your performance and choke! NOT ON MY WATCH!

Likewise, you have to trust in your skills and to have faith in your preparedness for any moment. Panicking is never a good idea and will not help in any situation. If a patient recovering from heart surgery in the ICU suffers a cardiac arrest or if he or she begins to exsanguinate internally from a leaking suture line, my panicking, rushing, or raising a raucous by hollering and screaming at everyone will do nothing except incite further chaos and seal that patient's deadly fate. My grace under fire is all that stands between that patient and certain death. I know what needs to be done, and I just do it! Within a minute or two, I'll have the chest open, right there in the ICU, delivering open-heart massage and stabilizing the patient, as we make our way back to the O.R. to fix whatever it is that needs to be fixed. Alternatively, I may just rapidly connect the patient to a portable form of the heart-lung machine, known as extracorporeal membrane oxygenation (ECMO) to get the patient stabilized. I'll confidently do whatever it takes to save his or her life without any hesitation! I know I got this! I have honed my lifesaving technical skills over the course of several years and thousands of repetitions, precisely for these and other moments just like it! Kind of sounds like Liam Neeson's character in the movie *Taken*, when he's warning his daughter's abductors about his "very particular set of skills; skills ... acquired over a very long career." I, too, am built to handle these challenging moments!

I refuse to allow fear of failure, fear of a bad outcome, to deter me from what needs to be done to save someone's life. There are no sure bets or guarantees for a successful outcome in heart surgery. The only thing that's for certain is death and taxes. With every surgery comes a finite risk of death, and with every patient comes a unique combination of risk factors that can influence the likelihood for an adverse event. The key distinction to keep in mind is that risk factors do NOT equate to contraindications. If the patient is a Jehovah's Witness (JW), for instance, like one of my recent patients, any perioperative bleeding whatsoever could be fatal, because that patient's religious beliefs preclude acceptance of any blood transfusions. So be it—are we to withhold lifesaving surgery for fear of what could go wrong, when not operating will lead to certain death? Mindful of the risks, I went ahead and performed a triple bypass operation on this patient, and he walked out of the hospital in a week.

In a heart transplant, if I were to wait around for the "perfect" donor heart to come along, the sure thing, all of our patients would die on the waiting list. It's impractical and obtuse to be addicted to certainty in any aspect of your life.

The same applies in this context. There's no such thing as a perfect heart, only the "right" heart for the "right" patient at the "right" time! It's a judgment call I have to make, usually in the middle of the night, for all the marbles, with someone's life hanging in the balance! It's a decision I have to own and to stand by. But, despite all that's at stake, I approach every challenging case with my "COTE of armor," as highlighted in the book *Performing Under Pressure*—Confidence, Optimism, Tenacity, Enthusiasm. That's what living *the Heart Way* is all about. It means choosing NOT to live in fear, to never shy away from the taking the game-winning shot.

Are you ready to finally get the proverbial monkey off your back? Are you tired of fear suffocating your ingenuity and potential? If so, where do you start? I'd say step one is making the conscious decision to break the invisible chains of bondage that fear has imposed on your life. Through subterfuge and intimidation, fear of failure has hijacked your mind somewhere along the way, holding your thoughts perpetually hostage. Left unchecked, this internal terrorist will squelch any hope or aspiration for living a life worth living and will steer you on a path towards mediocrity, even self-destruction. The good news is that you can end this captivity, once and for all. It's a choice!

In the real world, we don't negotiate with terrorists, nor do we give them a platform to expand their toxic program of hatred upon innocent civilians. So why would you ever negotiate with the terrorist that's in your head, whose main objective is to sabotage your life? Don't give fear the time of day. Be the person you're capable of becoming. Go about your business, holding your head high. If you need professional help, such as a therapist or psychiatrist, to get you over the hump, don't be bashful about it! Do what you need to get where you want, and don't worry about the he-said, she-said nonsense. People love to talk a big game or to critique someone else's. But rarely do they walk the walk or have the guts to even try. That's what big-time players and Cleaners do. That's what I wish for you.

As I've mentioned previously, it won't be all rainbows and unicorns along the way. There will be dark days, and you will occasionally fail. "I enjoy failure," said no one ever! That's okay. Pick yourself up, dust yourself off, and move on. You'll be better for it the next time around. You learn and grow from your mistakes and failures. No major league hitter has ever batted a 1,000. In fact, the best hitter in major league baseball history, Ty Cobb, averaged just over 0.360 over his twenty-four-year professional career. That means he struck out nearly two-thirds of the time at bat—doubtful he ever felt sorry for himself after an unsuccessful outing or admitted defeat. You do the same! Have the courage and fortitude to get back in and take your shot when the next opportunity presents itself. It happened for me, and it can also happen for you. The time will come when you also fearlessly crave the ball when the game is on the line. Regardless of where it is that you wage your battle for success, seize every moment that comes your way, and show the world who's boss! Own your life, because you've got this!

"Make the sting of
failure your triumphant
prologue."
–Brian Lima

CHAPTER 10

THE *HEART* SELL ON ENTREPRENEURSHIP: ALWAYS BE CLOSING

"I would like to be remembered as someone who did the best she could with the talent she had."—J. K. ROWLING, AUTHOR OF THE HARRY POTTER NOVELS

"I never dreamed about success. I worked for it."
—ESTEE LAUDER

Backed by their astounding records of success, Rowling's and Lauder's statements exemplify the essence of the hustler's spirt. They're testaments to what's possible when you live *the Heart Way* and you methodically apply all the lessons we've discussed throughout this book. This brings us to the one missing piece we haven't formally covered yet, something I didn't appreciate until well into my thirties, just as I finished serving my ten-year prison term—I mean, surgical *training*. Before I spill the beans on that, you're probably wondering why it took so long—this final lesson, that is, not the training. But that's just it, because my training WAS my life, devoted entirely to getting in all those critical reps, accruing 10,000 hours of practice, honing my craft, and developing that final polished product.

The telling of that story is what's occupied most of the pages in this book. I was like a mad scientist, cooped up in my own little bubble and consumed by my alchemical quest to become a magnum opus in my own right! Only later would I realize that not even a magnum opus "sells itself" in the real world. The reality is that, to make something of yourself in this world, you have to successfully market your brand. That's the cornerstone of entrepreneurship and the primary lesson I'd like to share in this chapter.

My critically acclaimed writing aside (kidding, obviously), our journey together has been pretty boring, if we're being brutally honest with one another. Sure, we've shared some laughs and perhaps shed a few tears along the way, but we haven't traveled very far at all. You see, for the entirety of this sojourn, we've just been touring the *Research & Development (R&D) Laboratories of **Brian Lima, Inc.*** (BLI). For the narcissist in me, BLI has quite a cool ring to it! But don't let the fancy name fool you, however. BLI is a far cry from the sprawling facilities of Apple Park, Google campus, or that of any other Fortune 500 company. BLI may sound "state-of-the-art," but it's really just a small-time, mom-and-pop operation working in relative anonymity.

This whole time, we haven't ventured beyond the heavily guarded borders of BLI headquarters to explore the wild blue yonder. Before this book, and up to this point in my life, I, admittedly, wasn't forthcoming with my intellectual property, and I remained completely engrossed with building the best *product* I could! The product, of course, was me, and my hands were full, juggling the responsibilities of chief architect, chief engineer, and chief executive officer of the BLI enterprise. Conspicuously absent from my business model was any marketing division or advertising efforts. I simply never bothered adopting such "ploys for attention." At least, that's how I used to regard such exertions. I've always been a strong believer that actions speak louder than words and that tacky self-promotion was the hallmark of insecurity. Unbeknown to me, this was a decidedly amateurish blunder on my part and would later come back to bite me. Like it or not, we all have to sell ourselves to be successful.

Now here we are, sans any nondisclosure agreement (NDA), and I'm an open book, sharing all of my company's deepest and darkest secrets. You've gotten to hear all about the blood, sweat, and years that went into product development. You've witnessed the evolution of a labor-intensive manufacturing process fueled with homegrown raw materials. I've regaled you with the all the maddening details, the exhaustive pursuit for quality improvement and enhanced efficiencies. And, finally, after several iterations and tweaks, it came time to bring this product to market. The time seemed right for my product launch. I could firmly attest to the dependability, the high quality, the resilience, and the moral character of this battle-tested war machine. It was top of the line, with all the bells and whistles, standing head and shoulders above the competition. So, like a new addition to the Harry Potter Series, the Brian Lima brand should sell itself, right? Fly right off the shelf? Fine; I'll stop annoyingly referring to myself in this quasi-third person now, but the answer here is obvious—not even close!

For starters, the notion that I'm a "top-shelf" brand is not a statement of fact and is completely open to debate. I'm just confident in my abilities and believe in myself, as should everyone. My track record speaks for itself, and I've rightfully earned a shot at breaking into the big leagues. Nevertheless, no matter how exceptional or highly sought-after any given product is, nothing actually "sells itself." Rowling's Harry Potter books or the next iPhone may very well sell out in minutes, but that's because they're established brands that have already won over the masses. They are known commodities and have garnered tremendous clout and media attention. The fact of the matter is that billions of dollars are spent in advertising campaigns and commercials for the hottest items on anyone's wish list. Look no further than the Super Bowl, where a thirty-second commercial will run over $5 million. No expense can be spared, when it comes to promoting your brand.

One way or another, you have to get the word out about how great your brand is, or else few will bother to give you the time of day. It's about hustling, giving the hard sell, pounding the pavement, weathering the ups and downs of the market or your field of interest, and never letting up. With rare exception, all successful entrepreneurs you'll meet will have endured countless failed business ventures and financial woes before finally catching their big break and closing on that one lucrative deal that nets them the mother lode. They didn't allow all their previous failures and rejections to deter them from staying on course and from angling for the next sales pitch.

Salesmanship is an art and may not come naturally for

most of us. In its most elemental form, where you eat only what you kill, the stress and the ruthlessness of this cutthroat existence can be overwhelming. If you want to catch a good glimpse of how brutal things can get, you need to check out the 1992 film, *Glengarry Glen Ross*. Right at the onset of the movie, Alec Baldwin's character delivers an epic seven-minute rant to a group of underperforming real estate agents. He viciously mocks their lack of moxie and killer instinct, when it comes to closing on a sale. Throughout the cruel invective, he repeatedly points to what he's listed on a blackboard, stressing the essence, or "ABCs," of salesmanship—"Always Be Closing!" Riddled with profanity and expletives, his tirade, to some, may seem obnoxious, offensive, and far from motivational. It's safe to say that you could never get away with such antics today—by thirty seconds in, the PC police would have forcibly subdued him and led him away in handcuffs! But if you can get past the vulgarity, the mantra, *"Always Be Closing,"* is not only at the core of salesmanship; it's at the very heart of entrepreneurship and success in general. It's about constant hustle and how to become the best possible version of yourself. Continually developing and optimizing your "brand" *IS* living *the Heart Way*, an imperative to be triumphant in any field or walk of life!

It wasn't until very recently that the concept of being an entrepreneur would have any real place or relevance in my life. After all, I'm a heart surgeon, and business acumen was not my strong suit. I stayed in my lane, as it were, sticking with what I knew and what I had devoted so much of my life to, as simple as that. Money just wasn't a driver for me, and I didn't factor it into my calling. And, for as long as I can remember, the term "entrepreneurship" conjured visions of sleazy

Wall Street tycoons in tailored suits brokering shady business deals in their fiftieth-floor corner office, as they sip on single-malt scotch. Think of Leonardo DiCaprio in the critically acclaimed *Wolf of Wall Street* flick. No thanks!

Such caricatures, I thought, operated solely on the fringes of our business and financial sectors, where the "bottom line" is often the be-all and end-all. There's no way that sort of stuff would ever rear its ugly head in health care, right? Wrong, again! "Health care has become corporatized to an almost unrecognizable degree," as Danielle Ofri pointed out in a recent *New York Times* piece ("The Business of Health Care Depends on Exploiting Doctors and Nurses," June 2019). This should come as no surprise. Money makes the world go round. The same rules of engagement apply anywhere money exchanges hands. They span all sectors of our society, and health care is no less corruptible than other industries. Between Big Pharma, private insurance companies, large hospital chains, and what amounts to a multitrillion dollar business, health care is fertile ground for corporate greed and fraudulent business practices. While the cast of characters may be playing on a different stage—a hospital rather than the trading floor of a stock exchange, for instance—many are ruthlessly driven to achieve the same ends—financial gain.

That modern medicine was an unofficially official part of corporate America would have never occurred to me. Throughout all those years as a surgical trainee, I was never really exposed to the business or entrepreneurial side of medicine. There were the occasional encounters with disgruntled surgeons here and there, bemoaning the progressively bureaucratic leanings of hospital administration and admonishing me that "if they were me," they'd jump ship and get an

M.B.A. STAT! But these were largely few and far between, so I ignorantly dismissed them as disillusioned has-beens gone rogue. You have to remember that I was a man on a mission, possessed and indoctrinated to disregard such petty musings and to simply stay the course.

A business degree? Give me a break! Yet, on second thought, I would later wonder if they were onto something. Naively, I had always assumed that all I had to concentrate on was to be the best heart surgeon I possibly could be and to take great care of my patients. The rest would take care of itself—salary, promotion, patient referrals, and the like. The fantasy I had dreamed up during my residency was a scene lifted straight out of the movie *300*—a Spartan youth's glorious return to civilized society as a hoplite warrior, lauded for having endured years of the harshest training imaginable. Upon finishing all those years of training, I envisioned making a grand entrance to my new hospital workplace, greeted with drums rolling and trumpet fanfare, consummating the highly anticipated arrival of the greatest thing since sliced bread—God's gift to medicine! The flood gates would magically open, and my clinic and operating-room schedule would be jam-packed with cases and new referrals. If only that were true, my life would be a heck of a lot easier! Maybe that's just what I had to tell myself to keep me sane all those years. I was in for quite the rude awakening…

Let me save you the suspense. I arrived at my first job after training in very anticlimactic fashion, with little ballyhoo. My naïve assumptions aside, a hospital, it turns out, is like any other place of business that has to generate revenue to keep the lights on. Heart surgeon or not, I was just another hospital employee—i.e., another line on some bean counter's spreadsheet, where the revenue I generated would be counted against my salary to calculate my employer's ROI (return on investment)—was I worth what they were paying me?

And since when did all this business jargon become relevant to doing cardiac surgery? Believe me: it doesn't stop there. Everything we do as physicians, from seeing patients in our offices to performing minor bedside procedures and diagnostic tests, all the way to transplanting a heart, is assigned a predetermined number of relative value units (RVUs)—that's basically how the amount of our reimbursement is calculated. The more patients you see or procedures you do, especially really complicated procedures, the more RVUs you rack up, and the greater your potential salary or bonus becomes—I'm not making this up. That's right; believe it or not, somewhere along the way, a pencil pusher decreed that doing a heart-by-pass operation was worth x number of RVUs. This nickeling and diming, for lack of a better phrase, gives you an idea of just how monetized and corporatized health care has become.

Referrals? Don't even get me started! While I was certainly a legend in my own mind, the reality was that no one in the community knew me from Adam. The only "Brian Lima" anyone's ever heard of is the world-famous Samoan rugby player, nicknamed "The Chiropractor," on account of the backbreaking hits he regularly delivers to his opponents! Ouch! Google it, and you'll see I'm not kidding. The humbling reality was that I was a new and unknown commodity within the physician referral network and was still wet behind the ears, as far as the network was concerned. Why would cardiologists refer me to a patient for open-heart surgery? They've never heard of me and have been sending their surgical referrals to other very capable surgeons for years. Years? That's right! It takes most of my colleagues several years to build their practice and referral base. I know social media would have you thinking differently, but make no mistake—you don't become a household name locally or beyond overnight.

To break into any market in any industry, your product (or brand) must offer some distinct advantage, cost benefit, or unique level of service relative to the competition. Think of the disruptive innovation Uber unleashed on the taxi industry or Netflix's game-changing impact on cable television. What's your niche? How do you set yourself apart? In my field, a lot of it boils down to delivering concierge service to your patients and your referring physicians. When they need you, you're available, affable, and able. Do you recall the three As I had mentioned earlier? The customer is always right, if you expect to Always Be Closing!

Competition was stiff, so I had to prove myself to every single patient and medical provider that crossed my path in this uncharted territory. Effectively, they were the consumers, and I had to sell them on my professional services. Very quickly, I learned that, in order to drum up business, I was going to have to get out there and network, shake hands, and toot my own horn. As an aside, it would have been nice if my professors had taught me this in medical school. At any rate, my brand wasn't going to sell itself, so my grassroots outreach efforts included quite the dog-and-pony show, complete with flashy PowerPoint slides, business cards, and online marketing initiatives. I had to relentlessly market my brand and to embrace my entrepreneurial spirit. In other words, it dawned on me that I had to become a good salesman, if I had any hope of having a successful heart-surgery practice. I *always* had to be *closing*, and I don't mean just the chests of the patients I had opened to do their cardiac surgery, if you catch my drift!

Yes, it was this crash course in Business 101 that forced me to revisit the "Always Be Closing" mindset. There was much more to it than just a memorable scene from a cult classic movie. It was a way of life in itself. I increasingly directed more time and energy to learning about the business world, reading books and articles written by many of the thought leaders and prominent CEOs featured in *Forbes* magazine and the *Wall Street Journal*. One prevailing concept that stood out to me was the recurring references made to "branding" and its direct correlation with profitable ventures in the marketplace. The idea that each individual has his or her own brand, was also extremely eye-opening. One's "brand," as defined by David McNally and Karl Speak in their book, *Be Your Own Brand*, "is a reflection of who you are and what you believe, which is visibly expressed by what you do and how you do it."

But branding is just one of the many other tools wielded by successful entrepreneurs. I was surprised to find that many of the other key facets of entrepreneurship also figured very prominently in my own life's experiences. The more I read, the more I realized that it wasn't just about money or generating profits. It turns out that being an entrepreneur is entirely more about things like passion, courage, confidence, drive, grit, resolve, tenacity, resourcefulness, and creativity, just to name a few. It sounds like *the Heart Way* to me! Who knew? Maybe I was an entrepreneur after all!

Chances are that you're also an entrepreneur and just didn't know it yet, either. We'd all love to make the most of the cards we're dealt, but sometimes we get lost in the shuffle of daily life. It can be difficult to bounce back from defeat, failure, rejection, or whatever else life can throw our way. As Mike

Tyson said in a postfight interview, "Everyone has a plan until they get punched in the mouth." But fear not, because I'm in your corner and I've got your back!

Far from a business guru myself, I did a considerable amount of legwork to drill down the basic fundamentals of entrepreneurship, the "e" in *the Heart Way*. I focused the bulk of my efforts on those aspects most generalizable to everyday life and to the pursuit of success. For your reading pleasure, I've taken the liberty of codifying the most salient features into four sections, each intended to maximize the potential for success in your life. They've certainly proven useful in my life, and I hope they serve you equally as well in yours.

1. Pigeonholes are strictly for the birds

Never mind staying in your lane. Don't limit yourself or your choices by whatever preconceived notion you had of what success looks like! You never know what fate may have in store for you, so never pigeonhole yourself. Get out there, spread your wings, and fly! I never fancied myself a writer of books. Heart surgeons aren't supposed to write about nonheart-surgery stuff or to venture outside of health care. Yeah, tell that to Dr. Oz! And yet here we are, and whether this book becomes a best seller or no seller, I gave it my all, and I'm proud that I was able to pull it off—que sera sera. As we discussed in Chapter 9, too many of us have become so addicted to certainty that we've unwittingly sabotaged our true potential. We avoid risk, and we stick with the safe, cozy, and boring path of least resistance that serves only to keep us grounded. Many of us fail to realize that uncertainty is where the real magic happens! Uncertainty is "the environment in which you grow, experience new things, and produce new, unprecedented results," as author Gary John Bishop describes in his book *UNFU*K YOURSELF*. I couldn't agree more with this statement. Abandon the pursuit of absolute certainty, and, instead, approach every challenge with cautious optimism. I promise you'll be better off in the long run.

The universe reliably grants us two things: (1) just enough information to guide the next immediate step and (2) the unmistakable visual accuracy of hindsight! Never in a million years, as the meathead, blue-collar kid growing up Jersey, would I have ever imagined living in North Carolina (ending up at Duke University), Texas, or Ohio (Cleveland Clinic), yet each of these "deviations from the plan" were, in actuality, tremendous periods of growth and maturation, establishing contacts and friendships with individuals that would later become heavy hitters and thought leaders in my field of cardiac surgery. These stints greatly diversified my portfolio of life experiences, reshaping my convictions and career trajectory, and, of course, they allowed me to meet and brainwash—I mean, convince—my amazing wife to marry me. Left to my own devices, I'm certain I would have robotically plodded along the "path" I had predetermined, one inexorably biased by the flawed and immature foundation on which it was crafted, only to miss out on countless blessings and invigorating moments! As the saying goes, "You want to hear God laugh? Just tell Him your plan."

The reality is that you just have to roll with it and trust in your gut that the next step is the right move. You won't be the same person next year, next decade, or thereafter. Likewise, your value system, priorities, and preferences will undoubtedly change. What may perfectly suit a certain season of your life may be completely incompatible with another. As you're learning the landscape of a new industry, for example, you may initially want to plug into a well-established, well-oiled, high-throughput machine to get a hang of things. Later, however, as you earn your stripes and discover your mojo, you may want to venture out on your own to create your own legacy and to punch your own hole in the universe!

To bring it full circle, this is exactly how I arrived at my current position, as Director of Heart Transplantation Surgery at North Shore University Hospital, the premiere quaternary care hospital on Long Island. It was about three years ago, and my wife and I were settling comfortably into our Dallas life, having just purchased and remodeled a new home. I had successfully established a national reputation in the field of heart transplantation and mechanical circulatory support. At the yearly meeting of the International Society of Heart and Lung Transplantation, data from the research I oversaw was featured in over ten separate presentations. Clinically, I had helped establish one of the highest-volume heart-transplant and mechanical-heart-pump programs in the country.

Then, lo and behold, I received a fateful call from Dr. Alan Hartman, the Chair of Cardiac Surgery for Northwell Health, one of the largest health care systems in the United States and encompassing over twenty hospitals. I couldn't believe what I was hearing. I was being recruited to help start and lead the very first heart-transplant program on Long Island! Returning to the Northeast, close to where I grew up, was the furthest thing on my mind.

Of course, I felt extremely flattered and honored to be even considered for such an incredible opportunity. Close to 90 percent of all the existing heart-transplant programs in the United States have been around for several years, if not decades. Starting a heart-transplant program is a massive undertaking. Heart transplant is among the most highly scrutinized of all procedures in all of medicine. Programs are closely monitored by the federal government (the Centers for Medicare & Medicaid Services, CMS), as they should be, and they can be shut down if they fail to maintain high one-year survival rates. With elite and storied programs like Columbia and Mount Sinai in close proximity, the region is, arguably, one of the most competitive heart-transplant markets in the world. This once-in-a-career opportunity would take place under the glaring spotlight of New York City mass media, making it the ultimate high-risk, high-reward venture. But as Frank Sinatra sang in "New York, New York," "If I can make it there, I'll make it anywhere!"

When you add up the populations of Long Island (Nassau and Suffolk Counties) and the surrounding boroughs of Brooklyn, Queens, and Staten Island, we're talking about an enormous community of approximately 8 million people who, until now, have not had a heart-transplant center to call their own. Because the nearest centers were predominantly located in Manhattan, this presented a considerable logistical barrier to access for this highly specialized level of care. If you've ever been to New York City, I don't have to tell you how crazy the traffic is and how difficult it is to get from point A to point B, even if they're a short distance apart. Now just imagine if you're afflicted with advanced heart failure and can barely get around.

This was all very troubling to me. The recurring question that kept running through my mind was, "How could this be?" I cringed at the hardship these poor patients and their loved ones faced, having to make the arduous and expensive commute into the city, back and forth, just to even be evaluated for a possible heart transplant, not to mention all of the postoperative visits and care. Then there's also the very disturbing statistics related to heart transplantation in New York: it ranks dead last, fiftieth out of the fifty states in the United States, for wait-list times, heart donation, and transplant rates per capita. The take-home point that registered loud and clear with me was that advanced heart failure is vastly undertreated in the Northwell Health service area! This community deserves better.

With that, and for first time in my career, I felt a simultaneous moral and professional obligation. I had to seize this opportunity and help Northwell improve the access to advanced heart care on Long Island and beyond. You could call this my second aha moment, the first being the epiphany I had experienced while watching a surgical procedure for the first time back in college. I was made for this. All those years of training and experience at some of the leading centers in the world for cardiac surgery and heart failure care had prepared me for this moment. I was ready. Fast forward to the present day, and I'm ecstatic to report that we've successfully launched our heart-transplant program and have done over twenty to date. We held a press conference to share the great news with the community, accompanied by Long Island's first heart-transplant patient, Ms. Yvonne Fleming (picture below). She's become a spokesperson and an advocate for organ donation and heart disease awareness. We couldn't be prouder of her excellent progress. This is really just the beginning, and our team of devoted heart experts is poised to lead, not only locally but also nationally and internationally. Stay tuned!

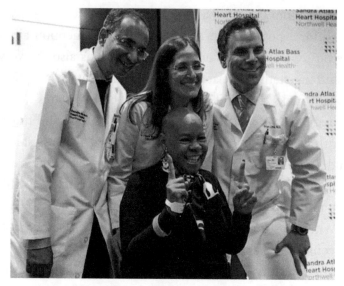

Press conference with our heart-transplant team (Dr. Syed Hussain, Dr. Gerin Stevens, and me) with our patient Ms. Yvonne Fleming, Long Island's first ever heart-transplant recipient!

2. No regrets allowed

Never second-guess decisions you made along the way that seemed like the correct move at the time! The should've's, would've's, could've's will drive you insane, if you let them. And, oftentimes, what may seem like a mistake or a wrong turn hasn't had enough time to manifest positively in your life yet. It's not to say you shouldn't learn from past errors and failures, but dwelling on them to the point that you lose your edge is pointless and self-defeating. Always keep your head high, own your past, cherish the present, and never bank on the future.

Life is precious, and it never affords you do overs. We all make mistakes, and some matter more than others. If you're like me, you're also probably harder on yourself than anybody else. I'm my own worst critic, and it takes a great deal of conscious effort to prevent negative self-talk from making an already bad situation even worse. No matter how bad things seem, you have to force yourself to remember that what's done is done. The past is in the past, so discipline your thought process so you don't keep reliving that awful or embarrassing moment. Focusing on the here and now when you're still aching from the sting of whatever that misstep was is the way you move on, grow, and improve. Say it out loud, talk yourself through it, and take control of how you will respond to the situation.

Whenever I lose a patient, it feels like a part of my soul is ripped out, and my head keeps spinning with a whirlwind of doubts, regrets, and intense grief. It's the worst feeling in the world, to know that you tried but failed to save someone's life, then to have to face the patient's family and to share in their unimaginable sorrow. I agonize over every decision, every move, and every single step I took before, during, and after the operation. Did I make the right decision to operate? Should I have waited for a better time when the patient was more stable? Could I have performed the operation technically any better? What did I miss?

I go through this debriefing ritual to extract whatever morsel of good I can from this tragedy, such as an instructive lesson on how to better approach a similar dilemma in the future. These are completely natural and understandable reactions, but letting them fester or snowball until I'm a panic-stricken mess is not okay. Not only is that a recipe for my own self-destruction; it's also an unacceptable disservice to my next patient, who's depending on my "A" game to save his or her life! I have a moral and a professional obligation to every single patient in my care, and I won't allow anything to interfere with it. Over the years, I've learned you have to just shut these mental traps down and to intently redirect yourself to the moment at hand. You have stay in tune with your thoughts and to practice mindfulness. Acknowledge what you're feeling and thinking in those difficult moments, but take over the reins when you sense that you're veering off course. Never relinquish control of your thoughts and emotions.

When things don't go according to the script, it may feel like your whole world is crumbling. But I hope you realize that you ultimately have the power to endure so much more than you think. You have your very own "jaws of life" that can extricate you from the haze of despair. It may take practice and time, even help from a professional, to help you harness that power. Have faith, and remember that everything happens for a reason. All those things that you never thought would occur, the detours, the tragedies, and setbacks—each one becomes an enriching part of your life. It is in those moments that you discover things about yourself you never knew. It's invaluable to go through these life lessons.

3. Invest in yourself, your "brand"

If you don't believe in yourself or feel certain that you're a sure bet, the real deal, how the hell could anyone else?! In retrospect, one of the earliest traces of my budding entrepreneurial spirit was convincing my dad to pay the astronomical $700 for a Princeton Review SAT prep course back in high school. This was a huge chunk of change for my factory-worker dad, but, boy, did it pay dividends. My scores subsequently skyrocketed several hundred points, earning me the necessary street cred to apply and to get accepted to a top college. Examples like this abound in my life, over and over again making sacrifices and taking calculated risks and delaying gratification, all in the relentless pursuit of becoming the best possible version of myself, building my brand!

All brands can become stale, irrelevant, or passé. To stay current, you must strive for continuous self-improvement. It's a well-known fact that the average CEO reads about sixty books per year. That's about a book per week, which is alarmingly impressive, given everything else that's on their plates. What about you? How many books do you read a year, or how many podcasts do you listen to? Maybe there's not enough time in your schedule for that kind of stuff, or so is that what you've been telling yourself?

You've listened to me describe, ad nauseam, how long and painful my surgical training was, but does that mean I'm free and clear now? No more learning for me? Of course not! My field is constantly evolving, and I need to, at a minimum, keep up or be leading the charge for innovation. I owe that to my patients and to myself. I subscribe to several medical journals that are relevant to cardiac surgery and heart failure. As part of my daily routine, I comb through the latest publications and studies so I can remain abreast of new technologies, surgical approaches, or outcomes from major clinical trials. If there's something new out there that I want to incorporate into my own clinical practice, then I go out and learn it!

But that just covers the clinical side of my professional identity. I'm also working towards an Executive MBA in Health Care Management, and I regularly read articles in the *Harvard Business Review,* the *Wall Street Journal,* and the like. I'm constantly reading books about how to be a better human overall, many of which I've cited in this book. So there's a lot of brand optimization happening over here at BLI—it never stops, and it keeps getting better!

Collectively, too many adults suffer from failure to thrive. In medicine, this terminology is used to describe a condition of delayed physical development secondary to inadequate nutrition. I'm applying it here to insinuate the apathetic state of stunted intellectual maturation that stems from chronic deprivation of mind-stimulating experiences. In his book *Own The Day, Own Your Life*, author Aubrey Marcus argues that when it comes to pathways for "human optimization," many of us are not making full use of our time or taking advantage of the "traveling university" that's right at our fingertips—our smartphones. As founder and CEO of Onnit, his company has broken new ground on holistic approaches to enhancing human performance across all aspects of our day-to-day existence. He attributes the success of his company to the foundational elements disseminated in his widely popular *Aubrey Marcus Podcast*, which continues to share a host of game-changing perspectives with all of its listeners.

There's a plethora of informative audiobooks and podcasts to choose from and to listen to during our commutes to and from work or at various points throughout our weekly schedule. "The point is to learn something," as Marcus emphasizes, "not gorge on nonsense," because "far too much media is designed to provoke and distract—the opposite of both mindfulness and mindfillness." His point is well-taken, and we'll address the downside of social media and time mismanagement in the following section. The goal we all should strive for is to make the most of our time, day in and day out, to end each day as better persons than we were the day before. It's never been easier to make that happen, so make better use of your time, and never settle for stagnation.

4. Your time matters, so use it wisely

As the clichéd expression "time is money" implies, time is a finite, limited resource we must strategically expend on a daily basis, balancing the needs and responsibilities within our personal and professional lives. To do this effectively, you must eliminate any and all distractions. I like to call this initiative "Stop the madness!" Don't become consumed by the mind-numbing and distracting haze of social media-induced stupor that has everyone in a trance and undermines the very fabric of the "hard work pays off" mantra I've been preaching throughout this book. It's staggering how preoccupied our society has become with celebrities and reality TV. Do yourself a favor and tune this nonsense out. If you're so caught up in the lives of these other people, what does that say about your life, or your brand? You're better than that! Rise above the nonsense! Ask yourself, "Why aren't the paparazzi tracking your every move?" It's time to put down your smartphone, roll up your sleeves, and get after it!

I know you're probably wondering how many pep rallies I can cram into one book. I may be a bit much, at times, but I promise that I'm much more mellow in person and that my heart's in the right place. In going that extra mile to drive my points across, I'm hoping to motivate and to inspire change, change that is much-needed in my not-so-humble opinion. The older I've gotten, the more concerned I've become about our society's progressively apathetic tendencies and about the wayward direction of our youth. Not enough of us have our heads in the game, so how can we expect the younger generations to fare any better? Instead, their heads are affixed to a smartphone screen, staring at click bait. And while I may not have kids of my own, you don't have to be a parent to recognize the troubling state of affairs among today's youth. It's not just me. A number of experts and authors have made their own keen observations in this regard. William Damon, for example, in his book *The Path to Purpose,* shares these startling results from studies he conducted:

> "Our initial findings reveal a society in which purposefulness among young people is the exception rather than the rule…only about one in five young people in the 12-22 year range express a clear vision of where they want to go, what they want to accomplish in life, and why."

Then there's Aubrey Marcus, whom I cited earlier, and his observations on smartphone trends:

> "Everywhere I go, I see people superglued to their devices. I see moms on their phones while their kids are screaming at each other…We are now a different species because of our devices. We are slaves to them. They own more of our attention than nearly everything else in our lives…Our phones have invaded our psyches…We've become enchanted, bewitched, seduced by the pull of the screen."

He recommends winding down our cell phone usage at the end of the day, to schedule periods of rest and meditative relaxation AWAY from our handheld technologies. More recently, at my alma mater Cornell University's New Student Convocation, Cornell President Martha E. Pollack urged the incoming students to "open your mind by freeing your ears."

This short quotation brilliantly sums up both the problem and the solution in a single breath. Her address hit the nail on the head, rendering a vivid snapshot of what modern-day life has devolved to:

> "As I drive in to work at Cornell every morning, I see dozens of students wearing these [earbuds] as they walk to class," she said. "They're all walking in the same direction, but they're not walking together. They're not listening to each other. Instead, they're listening to whatever is coming in through their headphones. The visual image is even more striking. They're saying, 'I am in my world, not the world around me; I am listening to someone else, not the human beings beside me.'" [http://news.cornell.edu/stories/2019/08/students-urged-connect-and-engage-without-headphones]

It seems that living and being present in the moment is a thing of the past. Everyone, everywhere, is glued to their phone. It's gotten out of control, and, like President Pollack, I'm urging you to free your mind and to take in the world around you. That's how you make the most of the cards you're dealt and how you live a life worth living—by doing it *the Heart Way!*

PART THREE

COLD *HEART* FACTS: JUST WHAT THE DOCTOR ORDERED

"I walk these streets
A loaded six-string on my back
I play for keeps 'cause I might not make it back
I been everywhere, still, I'm standing tall
I've seen a million faces
And I've rocked them all."
–Bon Jovi in "Wanted Dead or Alive"

"Your moment may come when you least expect it, so ALWAYS BE READY!"

–BRIAN LIMA

CHAPTER 11

STATE OF THE *HEART*: LIFE IN THE TRENCHES

*"Anyone who would attempt to operate on the heart
should lose the respect of his colleagues."*
—Theodor Billroth (1829–1894)

*"There are a hell of a lot of jobs that are scarier than live
comedy. Like standing in the operating room when a guy's
heart stops, and you're the one who has to fix it!"*
—Jon Stewart.

The human heart is quite the persnickety little organ and must be handled with tender, loving care, both figuratively and literally. In the case of the latter, just one false move, even the slightest of surgical miscues, and it's GAME OVER—checkmate! That's why I'd have to agree 100 percent with Jon Stewart's comical reference. Cardiac surgery *can* get pretty scary in a heartbeat (come on, I had to!). It's amazing to consider how far we've come in such little time, relative to other surgical specialties. Were he alive today, Dr. Billroth would also marvel at the phenomenal strides we've made in the field of cardiac surgery. Widely regarded as the founding father of modern abdominal surgery, Dr. Billroth was a master surgeon and the top dog of his day. He's credited with a number of "firsts," including the first successful gastrectomy (removal of the stomach) for gastric cancer, and he has a few surgical procedures named after him (Billroth I and II). But as his bold statement above denotes, no one dared trifle with the delicate heart back then—it was too dangerous to even contemplate in the nineteenth century.

That all changed in the latter half of the twentieth century, largely with the advent of the heart-lung machine, invented by the pioneering surgeon Dr. John Gibbon in the 1950s. By engineering this cardiopulmonary bypass circuit, he circumvented the major obstacle precluding successful heart surgery for all of preceding human history—instantaneous exsanguination and death the moment you make any incision on the heart! With this revolutionary machine, any blood that's shed in the operative field is brought back through the circuit and effectively recycled. This milestone development is what ushered in the modern era of cardiac surgery, where we routinely perform complex repairs or replacements of any part of the heart you can imagine. When all else fails, we can also just swap out the heart itself, giving the lucky recipient a fresh new lease on life, with a brand spanking new heart.

Now please bear with me, as I proceed to completely geek out on the area of medicine I'm most passionate about, the rapidly evolving field of advanced heart failure. And, just to reiterate, by "advanced," I'm referring specifically to end-stage heart failure, where the only fix is some form of "heart-replacement therapy," be it a transplant or a mechanical substitute. In the next chapter, we'll delve further into some of the statistics related to how alarmingly prevalent heart failure has become. For now, I want to give you a succinct overview of how I surgically tackle these challenging cases and a brief glimpse of what my life is like behind the scenes. As always, I'll try my darndest to make it entertaining!

We begin with the human heart and revisit what it is that makes this little dynamo such an indispensable and life-sustaining force—flow, *blood* flow, to be exact. A key player in the blood game is *heme*, an iron-containing molecule that avidly binds oxygen and transports it to the areas that need it the most. So blood flow is like nature's very own Amazon *Heme*, an ingenious way of repackaging the oxygen we inhale through our lungs and getting it delivered to our entire body faster than you can press the "Buy now with 1-Click" button on your Amazon app! Not to be outdone, this delivery service also includes a convenient return policy. All of the body's unwanted carbon dioxide is automatically picked up at no extra charge and rerouted back to the fulfillment center (the lungs) for exhalatory reprocessing—thereby feeding all the green plants on Earth via photosynthesis.

As long as the heart continues to deliver adequate blood flow to the rest of the body, everything remains copacetic. How much flow are we talking? Anywhere between four-to-eight liters every minute (l/min), give or take, depending on body size and level of exertion. For example, four l/min is plenty of juice to power those thenar muscles (of your thumb) for hours on end of scrolling pleasure on your smartphone. Conversely, you may need the eight l/min or more if you have to take the stairs at work because the elevator is broken. I count myself in that lot, as well. But if, at any point, your heart cannot meet the blood-flow demands of your body, then your physiologic state of nirvana goes to hell in a handbasket. Picture drowning, or suffocating—you're not getting enough oxygen. That's heart failure in a nutshell. Short of *curing* whatever it is that's ailing the heart in these instances or of replacing the heart itself, this unsustainable state of asphyxiation is uniformly lethal.

But what if we could jury-rig a plumbing workaround to reestablish normal blood flow? Bingo! Borrowing from the success achieved with the heart-lung machine, many of its core elements have been recapitulated into various strategies for mechanical circulatory support (MCS) outside the operating room and for extended durations of time. The impetus for the proliferation of these temporary and durable MCS modalities is the limited supply of donor heart organs available to save the exponentially growing number of patients with advanced heart failure. You may recall me touching on the crisis of donor-organ shortages back in Chapter 6. Nearly 11,000 Americans will die on the transplant waiting list this year alone. [www.nytimes.com/2019/06/11/opinion/organ-transplant-deaths.html]

For the estimated 300,000 people in the United States with advanced heart failure, only 1 percent, or about 3,000, of them end up getting heart transplants. What's more, the numerator hasn't budged much over the last couple of decades, while the denominator continues to swell at an alarming rate. For whatever reason, we haven't been able to appreciably expand our donor heart pool or overall number of heart transplants for some time. As a result of this supply-and-demand crisis, we've witnessed a veritable "rise of the machines" over the last decade, with a steadily increasing number of left ventricular assist devices (LVADs) being surgically implanted into patients as a bridge to eventual transplantation (BTT) or as a permanent cardiac substitute (destination therapy, DT) for those patients deemed ineligible for heart transplant. Former Vice President Dick Cheney was supported with his LVAD for almost two years, before finally receiving a heart transplant.

Speaking of famous people, you may be surprised to know that, in the early 2000s, one of the true giants in the burgeoning field of LVAD therapy was none other than Dr. Mehmet Oz. You may have heard of him, or you may have watched his wildly popular *The Dr. Oz Show*, winner of nine *Daytime Emmy Awards*! Well prior to his meteoric rise to celebrity superstardom, he was a leading international authority on cardiac transplantation and MCS and ran a highly successful research laboratory at Columbia. As a matter of fact, I came very close to working as a research fellow in that lab to fulfill my two-year research obligation during my Duke surgery residency. I was going to follow in the footsteps of one of the Duke senior residents who had just worked with Dr. Oz and who had a very productive experience in his laboratory.

I exchanged a few emails with Dr. Oz about my interest in working with him, but I eventually decided to stay put at Duke, mainly for logistical reasons. Who would've ever thought that Dr. Oz would go on to become an überfamous daytime talk show host? But, in the end, I was at least able to engage in a collaborative research effort with him, compiling LVAD data collected from both Duke and Columbia, to study the impact of LVAD therapy on subsequent heart-transplant outcomes. Along with Dr. Oz and other investigators from both institutions, I was the lead author of the 2006 article entitled "Does a Pre-Left Ventricular Assist Device Screening Score Predict

Long-Term Transplantation Success? A 2-Center Analysis," published in *Heart Surgery Forum* (shown below). This was by no means an earth-shattering contribution to the heart failure literature, but our findings, nevertheless, substantiated the practice of using LVADs as an effective bridge to heart transplant.

The Heart Surgery Forum #2006-1063
9 (5), 2006 [Epub July 2006]
doi:10.1532/HSF98.20061063

Online address: http://cardenjennings.metapress.com/link.asp?id=112496

Does A Pre–Left Ventricular Assist Device Screening Score Predict Long-Term Transplantation Success? A 2-Center Analysis

Brian Lima, MD,[1] Aftab R. Kherani, MD,[1] Jonathan A. Hata, MD,[1] Faisal H. Cheema, MD,[2] Jennifer Casher, BA,[2] Mehmet C. Oz, MD,[2] Vivek Rao, MD, PhD,[3] Jennifer M. Fal, BA,[2] Jonathan M. Chen, MD,[2] Jeffrey A. Morgan, MD,[2] Deon W. Vigilance, MD,[2] Mauricio J. Garrido, MD,[2] Carmelo A. Milano, MD,[1] Yoshifumi Naka, MD, PhD[2]

[1]Department of Surgery, Duke University Medical Center, Durham, North Carolina; [2]Department of Surgery, Columbia University, College of Physicians & Surgeons, New York, New York, USA; [3]Department of Surgery, University of Toronto, Toronto, Ontario, Canada

ABSTRACT

Background. A risk factor summation score was previously validated to successfully predict survival after insertion of a left ventricular assist device (LVAD). We investigated whether this scoring system also predicts clinical outcomes after eventual heart transplantation in LVAD recipients.

Methods. A retrospective review was performed on 153 consecutive patients who received an LVAD as a bridge to transplantation at 2 large-volume centers from 1996 to 2003. The scoring system was used to designate low- and high-scoring groups.

Results. Thirty-day mortality and 5-year survival after transplantation were equivalent between groups (4.46% versus 7.32% and 76% versus 70%, respectively). No difference was seen in length of posttransplantation ventilator dependence (2.83 ± 0.49 versus 3.3 ± 0.72 days) or intensive care unit monitoring (6.38 ± 0.77 versus 6.97 ± 1.1 days). However, low-scoring patients had a significantly decreased duration of inotrope support (5.57 ± 0.45 versus 7.74 ± 1.0 days, $P = .035$).

Conclusion. A risk factor summation score may predict which LVAD patients will require prolonged inotropic support following heart transplantation. However, survival in high-risk (elevated score) LVAD patients following heart transplantation is comparable to low-risk groups, favoring the continued practice of LVAD implantation as a bridge to transplantation even in high-risk patients.

INTRODUCTION

Left ventricular assist devices (LVADs) have become a standard therapeutic strategy to bridge patients with end-stage heart failure to transplantation [Peterze 2002; Kherani 2004]. Despite an increasingly critically ill population in

Received May 18, 2006; accepted June 2, 2006.

Address correspondence and reprint requests to: Brian Lima, MD, Cardiothoracic Surgery Research Fellow, Division of Cardiovascular & Thoracic Surgery, Duke University Medical Center, DUMC Box 3043, Durham, NC 27713, USA; 1-919-672-3143; fax: 1-919-684-8563.

which they are used, the majority of patients undergoing LVAD implantation survive to eventual heart transplantation, and long-term survival may be superior to that of medically managed recipients [Aaronson 2002]. However, controversy remains regarding the optimal timing and patient population in which to perform transplantation after LVAD placement [Gammie 2004].

In 1995, Oz et al developed a scoring system for LVAD recipients to facilitate patient selection and better predict those who would benefit from this intervention [Oz 1995]. As LVAD technology became more advanced and their use was expanded to sicker patients, the scoring system was revised in 2002 to more accurately reflect these changes [Rao 2003]. This scoring system has demonstrated the ability to accurately predict mortality following LVAD implantation. What remains to be seen, however, is whether sicker patients (with higher scores) have comparable survival and morbidity to those with lower scores after undergoing eventual heart transplantation. Addressing this question is the goal of this study.

METHODS

One hundred fifty-three LVAD recipients who underwent cardiac transplantation at 2 institutions, New York Presbyterian Hospital and Columbia University (September 1996-May 2002) and Duke University Medical Center (May 1996-May 2003), were included in this study. The length of follow-up ranged from 456 to 2987 days, with a mean of 1405 days.

The LVAD scoring system currently is based on a scale of 10 points, with an inverse relationship between score and clinical stability [Rao 2003]. At the time of LVAD implantation, 4 points are assigned if the patient is ventilated, 2 points if the implantation is performed in the setting of postcardiotomy shock, 2 points if the patient already has an extracorporeal LVAD in place, 1 point if the central venous pressure is greater than 16 mmHg, and 1 point if the prothrombin time exceeds 16 seconds. Each patient in this study was assigned to one of 2 groups. The highly scored group (group H) comprised patients with pre-LVAD scores in the range of 6 to 10. The lower-scored group (group L) included patients with scores of 0 to 5.

When it comes to LVADs, it's important to bear in mind that, instead of replacing the heart, an LVAD is surgically attached to the heart. It takes over the workhorse function of the left ventricle, the main pumping chamber of the heart that delivers blood to the entire body (see image below). The main drawback is that it's powered by special external batteries tethering the device via a "driveline," or power cord, that traverses the abdominal wall. This means that an LVAD patient cannot submerge in water but can still take regular showers as long as the driveline exit site is appropriately shielded or covered. But LVAD patients otherwise enjoy an excellent quality of life and can pretty much do anything else, including exercise and travel, not to mention being ALIVE, to share quality time with their loved ones.

While the first-generation LVADs were rather sizeable and somewhat clunky, the most recent devices in clinical use are extremely sleek, efficient, and less prone to device malfunction or adverse events, such as clot formation or strokes. I'm extremely proud to have been one of the principal investigators for the multicenter MOMENTUM 3 trial that studied the newest LVAD approved for human use, the HeartMate 3™. The unprecedented results we observed in this landmark trial led to its relatively speedy approval by the FDA for all clinical indications. For the first time, an artificial heart pump was shown to have results on par with heart transplantation, heralding a monumental leap forward for the field. [www.nejm. org/doi/full/10.1056/NEJMoa1900486]

Aside from LVADs, which offer a durable solution for patients with end-stage heart failure, an assortment of short-term MCS options have also been devised to stabilize "crashing and burning" patients that are far too unstable for big

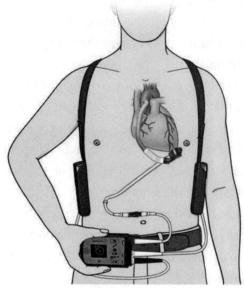

Schematic illustrating a prototypical LVAD (left ventricular assist device) used to treat patients with advanced heart failure that is refractory to medical treatments and not amenable to conventional heart-surgery procedures. This mechanical heart pump is surgically implanted and powered by external batteries attached to a power cord that's brought outside of the body from inside the chest.

open-heart procedures. Some may be dying before your eyes and are requiring CPR (cardiopulmonary resuscitation), because they're unresponsive or they're in full-blown cardiac arrest. In these moments of desperation, the only available trick up our sleeves is urgently connecting the patient to a portable form of the heart-lung machine known as ECMO (extracorporeal membrane oxygenation). This entails quickly gaining access to a major peripheral artery and vein, such as the femoral vessels located in the groin region, and inserting cannulas (long hoses about the width of your finger) into

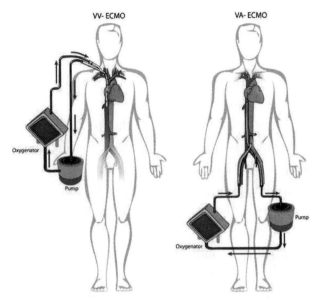

Portable heart-lung machine circuit known as ECMO (extracorporeal membrane oxygenation) can be used to provide complete heart and lung support (VA, venoarterial) or only lung support (VV, venovenous). The tubing for the circuit is inserted directly into large peripheral arteries and veins, as shown. [From Squiers, J. J., Lima, B., and DiMaio, J. M. "Contemporary Extracorporeal Membrane Oxygenation Therapy in Adults: Fundamental Principles and Systematic Review of the Evidence. The Journal of Thoracic and Cardiovascular Surgery, July 2016]

them, to create a circuit of blood flow that's propelled by an external pump (see figure below). The deoxygenated (low in oxygen, high in carbon dioxide) blood leaving the body via the vein cannula passes through an oxygenator (which adds oxygen and removes carbon dioxide) before returning to the body through the arterial cannula.

The trick, of course, is getting someone on ECMO support as soon as possible, because the risk of irreversible brain damage skyrockets the longer someone is requiring CPR. That's why it's never a dull day in my neck of the woods, because you never know what you're in for. Like the calm before the storm, I'm always a bit wary when things are too quiet. The next thing you know, the CODE BLUE alarm goes off overhead, and it's off to the races…

Putting patients on ECMO, as they're actively undergoing chest compressions, makes it very technically challenging and fraught with risk, such as internal bleeding or erroneously accessing the artery when you're going for the vein, and vice versa (normally, arterial blood is bright red, and venous blood is dark blue, but when someone is coding, blood will look equally dark in both veins and arteries). For that reason, I'm a big proponent of immediately transporting the patient to the cardiac catheterization lab, where we can use live X-ray visualization, to ensure we're inserting these cannulas into the desired locations. We've gone to great lengths to streamline and to protocolize this process, believing that the added accuracy and safety of this strategy is well worth the extra couple of minutes required to transport the patient to the optimal procedural setting.

ECMO also comes in handy in a variety of other scenarios, such as worsening shock from a major heart attack or lung failure in patients with severe flu or chronic lung disease, despite their being on a ventilator with maxed-out settings. Sometimes, at the conclusion of an open-heart surgery, the heart can't be weaned off the heart-lung machine—it simply won't take off on its own, and you need a rescue strategy. I've gotten many a frantic SOS call from colleagues stuck in the O.R. with their patients, following multiple failed attempts at separating them from the cardiopulmonary bypass machine. Perhaps the heart was a bit weak, to start with, or the procedure was very involved, and the heart was kept still way too long. Whatever the reason, ECMO can safely bail you out of the O.R. and give the heart a few days to recover. All it involves is switching over from the existing circuit to the portable ECMO machine and letting the dust settle before making the next move.

Along with ECMO, another class of temporary support devices, known as percutaneous VADs, has emerged over the last decade (see figure below). Basically, these devices are miniaturized pumps each mounted on a catheter and deployed

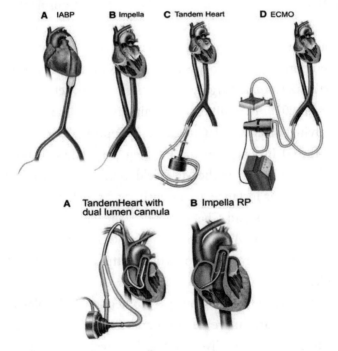

Contemporary, commercially available percutaneous left- (upper panel) and right- (lower panel) ventricular mechanical support devices. ECMO indicates extracorporeal membrane oxygenation; and IABP, intra-aortic balloon pump. [Reproduced from Circulation: Cardiovascular Interventions. 2017]

under X-ray or ultrasound (echocardiography) guidance. They're basically *VADs-on-a-stick*. The neat thing about them is that they can selectively support one side of the heart (left, LVAD; right, RVAD) or the other, or both, depending on the level of support required. They can be utilized in conjunction with ECMO as an adjunct to prevent overdistention of the heart chambers—long story, the details of which are beyond the scope of this chapter. More important, any of these temporary MCS tools are intended as a short-term (weeks) bridge to either recovery of the heart itself or to definitive treatment with a surgically implanted LVAD or a heart transplant.

I've written and researched quite a bit in the MCS space, and, most recently, I coauthored a chapter entitled "Temporary Circulatory Support Devices" for the upcoming textbook *Cardiac Surgery: A Complete Guide*, set for publication in 2020. In addition, I remain an active member of the Evolving Mechanical Circulatory Support Research Group (EMERG) Investigators, exchanging ideas and collaborating with other leaders in the MCS field to help advance it further. Last year, for instance, we published an article reviewing the "Controversies and Challenges of Ventricular Assist Device Therapy" in the *American Journal of Cardiology*, with me as the lead author (Link to article: https://doi.org/10.1016/j.amjcard.2018.01.034).

Together we're doing our part to help meet the global epidemic of heart failure head-on and to maximize our capacity to save as many lives as possible. Technical refinements in MCS technology will undoubtedly improve the outcomes of these therapies and will foreseeably supplant the need for heart transplantation altogether. Whatever happens, one thing is for certain: the future is bright for this field, promising a beaming ray of hope on the horizon for heart failure patients. It's immensely satisfying and motivating to know that, on some level, I will have played a role, albeit small, in seeing these hopeful aspirations come to fruition.

I feel incredibly fortunate to be an active, contributing member to this field of cardiac surgery. It was a long, long, long (did I mention "long"?), hard-fought journey to make it this far, but well worth all of the blood, sweat, and years. It's all the more satisfying when I think of all those exasperating inquiries I had to endure from skeptical friends and family along the way or when I caught wind of the disparaging comments they were muttering about me behind the scenes. "So are you like still in school? What's taking so long? Are you ever going to finish? 'So-and-so' is already out in practice, and they started med school way after you? Brian's been at this forever...is he even a doctor yet?"

It's a cruel world, and people often mock that which they don't understand. I never let the naysayers get me down. They fueled my drive, as I've attested to throughout this book. Every now and again, I'll catch myself having a split-second out-of-body experience, observing myself there in the zone performing open-heart surgery from the vantage point of that timid, chubby kid growing up in a Cuban immigrant household. The younger "me" is completely blown away by what he's witnessing, and the current "me" can't help smiling widely underneath my surgical facemask. I really made it! I'm living my American Dream and doing what I truly love!

I never take any of it for granted. Every day is a gift! It's all gravy, baby! You could say that I'm a frequent flier on the cloud-nine express, and, most days, I am pinching myself to see if I'm dreaming. Granted, my sleep cycle, or lack thereof, and daily dose of stress would have many of you questioning my grasp of reality or level of sanity. There are certainly days that try my patience and that push me to the limits of my stress and fatigue tolerance. I may bend, but I never break, and I ALWAYS stay positive. There again, I say—I love my calling, the good, the bad, and the ugly! No, I'm not a glutton for punishment, but maybe I can't stop drinking the Kool-Aid. It's the exhilarating life in the trenches of a heart surgeon's breakneck existence! You either love it or hate it, but there's no in between.

Now, more than ever, it's become increasingly difficult to find those willing to sign up for the rough-and-tumble world of cardiac surgical training. Standing as the epitome of delayed gratification within the medical profession, a decade of training is a hard sell in a society consumed by instant gratification. It's not for everyone, to say the least. Every year, there are fewer and fewer applicants to heart-surgery training programs, plummeting by almost 50 percent over the last twenty years. When you factor in the projected growth of the elderly population and the surging rates of cardiovascular disease, most experts anticipate a cataclysmic shortage of able-bodied heart surgeons by 2035. Of course, from a supply-and-demand perspective, these projections paint a rosy outlook for my future job security. I fully expect to be operating well into my sixties, and maybe even beyond, if I can stay in shape. But, like global warming or any other looming crisis, these troubling trends should be cause for grave concern for the public at large. How will we ensure adequate access to advanced heart care in the future? What measures can we take now to increase our heart-surgery workforce?

One obvious place to start is to revamp the training

paradigm and to make it more palatable for potential applicants. Efforts to sweeten the deal and to attract more qualified candidates have gone so far as to truncate the period of
training from the insane decade that I weathered (seven years
of general-surgery residency, plus three years of a cardio-
thoracic-surgery fellowship) down to an integrated six-year
residency program known as I6. The drawback is that, with
significantly less time allotted for operating in the abdomen,
you could never emerge from an I6 program as a fully trained
general AND cardiothoracic surgeon. But, on the flipside, if
the final objective is to create a cardiac surgeon, does it make
sense to spend all that extra time doing umpteen gallbladder
removals and colon resections versus more high-yield reps in
procedures directly relevant to heart surgery? The answer is
obviously "no," and the overhaul of this time-honored surgical
rite of passage is long overdue. I wish such fast-track options
were available to me back when I was applying. This modifica-
tion is a welcome change, and it mirrors how, historically, heart
surgeons from overseas were trained for decades. The jury is
still out on what impact these changes will have on the quality
of the finished product, but, regardless, I welcome all the newbie graduates with open arms to the "dark side of the Force"!
I pride myself on playing well in the sandbox with everyone,
not to mention that we clearly need the reinforcements.

I've grown quite accustomed to the controlled chaos of my
profession. It's become my norm, and I couldn't imagine living any other way. The downside is that it's nearly impossible
for me to "leave work at the office." You can't simply turn it
"off" or clock in and out. Most of my clinical practice involves
taking care of the most critically ill heart patients, with hearts
so weak that we've exhausted all conventional medical and

surgical options. They need new hearts, or the next best things—mechanical substitutes, such as implantable mechanical pumps.

Their conditions can deteriorate rapidly and without warning, randomly progressing from relative clinical stability one minute to being in circulatory extremis the next. That's why there are a lot of "I'm sorry but's" that spring up regularly in my hectic routine. "I'm sorry honey, but it doesn't look like I'm going to make it to dinner tonight." "I'm sorry, but I have to cancel my dental appointment, because one of my patients is crashing." You get the picture…More often than I care to admit, my personal life or plans for leisure have to take a backseat to the chaotic and unpredictable world that is my calling.

Having devoted nearly an entire extra year of my heart-surgery training (tenth year), as well as the bulk of my clinical practice over the last seven years, to the surgical management of these advanced heart failure patients, I've acquired the requisite skill set and experience to meet their care needs. Their only fighting chance is being cared for by those who will battle constantly and exhaustively to the bitter end. Shift-work mentality has no place in my line of work, especially when it comes to heart transplant and the tricky business of fielding donor-heart offers from regional organ procurement organizations (OPOs).

The patients on our waiting list are desperately counting on me to make the right decision, to thoroughly evaluate every single donor-heart offer I get called about, and to come up with a winner. I may be sound asleep, but if that call comes in at 2:00 a.m., I have to spring into action, because now we're on the clock—you're only allotted one hour to accept or to decline an organ offer when your center becomes the "primary" one (the next one up on the list) for that donor organ. Given what's at stake, it's really not a lot of time, so you have to proceed as expeditiously as possible. I hop on my laptop, log on to the UNOS (United Network of Organ Sharing) portal, and fully vet the online donor-organ profile. By thoroughly combing through everything, from lab tests to functional studies and imaging, I can make the call—yay or nay—while my wait-listed patient's life hangs in the balance. The patient's time may be running out, so waiting until the next offer comes around may not be an option. This could be the last chance the patient ever gets, before something catastrophic happens and we lose our window of opportunity. I have to make every call count and to be certain that a "no" is really a no.

When we pull the trigger and accept a donor heart, the real drama begins to unfold, as our entire team is thrust into what feels like a real-life episode of the hit drama series *24*, where counterterrorism agent Jack Bauer has precisely twenty-four hours to save the world. In our case, the nerve-racking "tick-tock" of the clock is also reverberating loudly in our heads—it's a race against time to flawlessly procure the donor heart, to safely return it by air (jet or helicopter) or land (ambulance and sirens) to our recipient in the O.R., and to surgically implant it in under four hours. Why four hours? Relative to other transplantable solid organs, such as the kidney, which can reliably tolerate out-of-body times (cold ischemic times) of twenty-four hours and beyond, the heart is much less tolerant, with outcomes suffering beyond the four-to-six-hour mark. I'll go into that further later on in the chapter.

Led by another surgeon, the donor-procurement team travels to the donor hospital, which may be several hundred miles away from our hospital. Typically, I wait in the O.R. with our recipient, and when my partner tells me that he's visualized the donor heart and that it looks as good in person as it did on paper, we're a go—"the heart is good!" If the recipient is a "redo," i.e., has had previous heart surgery, such as an LVAD implant, then I have my work cut out for me, on account of all the scar tissue. Up to two-thirds of the transplants done these days are in patients bridged with an LVAD.

These are by no means enjoyable to revisit on the night of the transplant, presenting a formidable hornet's nest that must be approached with great care! Imagine a pulsating mass of thick scab, totally plastered to the overlying breastbone, with no recognizable anatomy. Think of excavating a fossil, except that it's moving and that if you veer off by just one millimeter with your dissection, someone can instantly bleed to death. Normally, for a "virgin" chest, it would take me less than twenty minutes to open a chest, connect to the heart-lung machine, and surgically excise the recipient heart (cardiectomy). In a tough redo, however, it could take me as long as two hours—and that's after innumerable reps and years of experience.

Heart transplant is like the ultimate team sport, so, to adhere to our four-hour rule, we must execute a precisely choreographed dance, down to the minute. My partner doing the donor-heart removal can have the heart out and be on his way back to us within thirty minutes. It takes me only about fifty-to-sixty minutes to sew in a new heart, so, in the interest of time, I'm ideally ready to start sewing the moment the donor heart arrives into my O.R., redo or not. This leaves approximately two-to-two and a half hours of "travel time," e.g., from the donor hospital to the airport, plus the flight time back here, and so on. Once the heart is in, it's a science and an undertaking in and of itself to (1) ease the new heart into its new home and (2) to get all the bleeding under control, especially if it was a tough LVAD-explant case.

The proof is in the pudding, and we'll know pretty readily whether the heart we selected is up to snuff! To add to the drama, no scenario is straightforward, because all donors under consideration, along with the potential recipients of their organs, have their fair share of undesirable characteristics, i.e., risk factors that must be weighed to hammer out the decision. That being said, you'd be astonished how often we've come across hearts that were declined by other centers but that turn out to be hidden gems upon closer inspection. By going the extra mile, examining every iota of data pertaining to that donor and occasionally requesting that certain tests be repeated, we've uncovered totally viable hearts that were overlooked by centers before us. They may have taken only a cursory glance and reflexively rejected the offer at the first hint of any potential deal breaker(s). These absolute contraindications are often quite subjective and are guided solely by anecdotal experience that is heavily biased and quite center-specific. Far greater than just semantics, the crucial distinction here cannot be overstated—risk factors do not automatically equate to contraindications, and areas of controversy abound in the science of recipient-donor matching.

There are innumerable variables that enter into the decision-making process. Maybe the heart wall is a little thicker than we'd like or the donor is a bit smaller than the recipient. All of these calculated risks need to be hashed out. Whenever I'm not entirely swayed one way or another, I'll frequently rouse a few of my team members from their slumber and convene an impromptu conference call. During this meeting of the minds, we pour over the data and render a team decision. Much more than some agonizing, team-building exercise in collective sleep deprivation, most of these wee-hour deliberations are centered on minimizing the risk of *primary graft dysfunction* (PGD), the most dreaded complication after any solid organ transplant and the leading cause of death in the immediate postoperative period. In PGD, the newly implanted heart inexplicably exhibits severe dysfunction that requires high doses of synthetic adrenaline medicine infusions or even escalation to ECMO support for stabilization. The heart may eventually recover over the course of a few days, but, in a perfect world, we'd prefer avoiding this ominous complication at all costs.

PGD has resided in my cross hairs for quite some time. It's the bane of my existence as a heart-transplant surgeon, and, for the last fifteen years, I've expended an inordinate amount of time and effort towards unraveling the PGD conundrum. When, by what all accounts *should* be a donor heart that immediately takes off like a locomotive in the recipient, instead stumbles feebly out of the gates, you can begin to understand why so many of us in the field are so heavily invested in this endeavor. It's a devastating and gut-wrenching feeling I'd prefer never to suffer through again. Of course, it also didn't help matters that until the International Society of Heart and Lung Transplantation (ISHLT) finally released their consensus statement in 2014, a universal definition or severity scale of PGD was sorely missing.

Armed with this new definition, I employed every available resource at my disposal, as the Director of Clinical Research in Heart Transplantation & MCS at Baylor University Medical Center, to create one of the largest and most comprehensive single-center heart-transplant databases. The massive UNOS and ISHLT registries of several thousand heart-transplant patients from all over the world lacked sufficient granularity to grade PGD. Our database, on the other hand, was intentionally designed to encompass all of the diagnostic criteria necessary to capture PGD and its severity. We combed it for every clue, every trend, and every clinical variable imaginable to home in on those factors that yielded the highest statistical probability for the development of PGD. In 2017, we were among the first groups in the world to validate the newly minted ISHLT criteria for PGD, and we published our findings in the *European Journal of Cardiothoracic Surgery*. [https://academic.oup.com/ejcts/article/51/2/263/2439479].

One of the principal findings of our analysis was that 30 percent of heart-transplant recipients experience some degree of PGD (mild—18 percent, moderate—4 percent, or severe—8 percent) and that the severity of PGD directly correlated with the risk of death during the first year. The mortality risk associated with "mild" PGD was negligible, and so it appeared that only moderate or severe PGD had any clinical relevance. With the help of our expert biostatistician, we were able to pinpoint a handful of risk factors that were highly predictive of moderate-to-severe PGD. To our surprise, absent from this list were the usual suspects identified in prior studies conducted back when we weren't all speaking the same language in the heart-transplant community and when wildly inconsistent criteria were used to designate PGD. Things like older donors or recipients, donor hearts with thicker walls (hypertrophy), or donor hearts with prolonged ischemic times (hearts kept out the body longer than four-to-six hours before implantation) didn't seem to be the main drivers of PGD.

No, what really stood out and what dramatically increased the likelihood of significant PGD in our patient cohort was an "undersized donor," meaning that the donor heart was too small to support the bigger recipient. This is the conceptual equivalent of putting the engine from a small car into an armored tank. So how can we bungle something as simple as size? That would intuitively seem like a gimme, right? But as far as size matching goes, the *officially* sanctioned methodology by the ISHLT was purely body-weight-based, with a general recommendation of not undersizing the donor by more than 30 percent.

The problem with using only body-weight calculation is that it fails to account for the variations in heart size that are attributable to gender, age, and height! All things being equal (age, height, and weight), the heart of a woman will be physically smaller than her male counterpart. Little did I know that sophisticated cardiac MRI studies have generated spot-on predicted heart-mass (pHM) calculations that incorporate all four of these variables (height, weight, age, and sex) into a simple equation. I learned about this development when I read the 2014 article "Cardiac Size and Sex-Matching in Heart Transplantation: Size Matters in Matters of Sex and the Heart" in the *Journal of the American College of Cardiology: Heart Failure.* The article caught my eye not only because of the witty double entendre in its title but also because it elucidated a plausible "smoking gun" in the PGD phenomena.

The study revealed that donors undersized by greater than 10 percent pHM had significantly increased risk of death. While it failed to mention anything about PGD as the underlying cause of death (PGD was not yet formally defined), it did raise the question as to whether we should consider using pHM rather than body weight for our size-matching calculations in heart transplant. My hypothesis was that the increased risk of death the study observed in patients receiving smaller donors (by pHM) was due to PGD. Fast forward three years later to our published study, where we demonstrated that undersizing donors by pHM, but *not* just by body weight, had a direct causal link to moderate-to-severe PGD. In a subsequent head-to-head comparison between body weight alone and pHM, published the following year in *The Journal of Heart and Lung Transplantation,* we again showed that pHM was predictive of PGD and should supplant body weight as the preferred method of size matching [https://doi.org/10.1016/j.healun.2018.03.009]. In fact, it had already become a standard part of my practice and of the way I size up, pun intended, all of my donor offers!

I'm happy to report that, on the basis of all of this work, pHM will be officially incorporated into the next edition of the ISHLT donor-selection guidelines and that I was invited to be one of the contributing authors. It's immeasurably rewarding to work so passionately towards a goal and have the fruits of your labor impact the greater good of the patients not only under your direct care, but also of the myriad heart failure patients across the world, hoping to eke out as much time as possible on this Earth, with a decent quality of life. To me, that's what's it's all about. That's what makes the crazy hours, the sleepless nights, and the constant stress all worth it! Never give up on your dreams, and always take the high road. I promise you everything else will work itself out in the long run! Just be true to yourself, and do you part!

"ALWAYS take the high road, no matter what WAZE is telling you. No shortcuts allowed. The HEART WAY is ALWAYS the right way."

–Brian Lima

CHAPTER 12

*HEART*WIRED FOR HEALTHY LIVING: YOUR BEST LIFE AWAITS

"Our bodies are our gardens – our wills are our gardeners."
—William Shakespeare

"To keep the body in good health is a duty, otherwise we shall not be able to keep our mind strong and clear."—Buddha

The journey to bring you this book has been a labor of love that I will always cherish. It started over six years ago, when I was abruptly awakened in the middle of the night with a flood of ideas that I feverishly scribbled out onto a notepad on my nightstand. The more I wrote, the more I kept dredging up, as though I had serendipitously tapped into some endless stream of consciousness. I know this sounds completely random! It certainly was, and, the next morning, I remember thinking, "What just happened?!" Even to this day, I can't really convey what exactly drove me to start this adventure, but I can tell you it was something that I couldn't let go, even as a young heart surgeon diligently working to grow my fledgling clinical practice. Whenever I had a spare moment, I would jot down more ideas and themes I wanted to include. As my repository of notes got bigger and bigger over the years, it took on a life of its own. It was an inescapable sense of obligation to share my story, to share the countless invaluable lessons I learned while chasing my American Dream. This cathartic process forced me to revisit and relive some of the most tragic and challenging moments of my life, but equipped this time around with a fresh perspective and a keen sense of gratitude for those trying times.

Those tough times are what molded me into the person I am today. For that I remain eternally grateful. I wouldn't trade places with anyone. Everything happened for a reason, and that reason, while virtually imperceptible at the time, in retrospect always comprised a key formative step in my development and maturation. I sincerely hope that the conceptual framework of *the Heart Way* I've outlined in this book can also enable you to push beyond your perceived limitations and to reach your full potential. At the end of the day, I truly believe that no matter what the world throws our way, we are the final arbiters of what impact that event, stressor, or circumstance will have on our lives. We get to decide to press on, regardless, *the Heart Way,* avoiding all shortcuts, always taking the high road, with eyes facing forward, affixed on the future and oblivious to the past, essentially becoming heart to beat!

All that being said, I'd be remiss if I didn't put my surgical cap back on for a moment and leave you with some essential clinical pearls to promote your overall health. After all, my true passion in life will always be found in the operating room, doing heart surgery. But, at the risk of limiting future business prospects, I'd prefer you avoid needing heart surgery, if at all possible. As I often say to friends, family, and former patients, "I hope to never see you in a professional capacity!" Not surprisingly, the feeling is usually mutual. If you're needing to see someone like me for heart care, it means you've crossed over into the realm of critical heart disease, and death may be right around the corner. That's *no bueno*! Think of me as the goal line defense in football, all that stands between you and the end zone less than a yard away—there I go again with another sports analogy. Since it's the last chapter, I promise it's the last one.

But, just like in football, allowing the offense to make it all the way to the one-yard line could have possibly been avoided. Mental errors, lapses in judgement, or poor effort more than likely precipitated the defensive collapse. Heart disease rarely just appears out of the blue, affording ample time and preventive measures to halt its progression. More important, apart from the heart being the most critically important organ (kidding, sort of; okay, not really), maintaining heart-healthy practices will cover your overall health and will maximize your lifespan. Heart health and living *the Heart Way* go hand-in-hand. As the quotations from Buddha and Shakespeare cited above imply, we can't lead productive, fulfilled lives without taking care of our health, our physical and mental well-being.

Also always remember that material possessions are replaceable, but you and your loved ones are NOT! Don't take your health for granted! Be thankful and appreciative of your good health—don't squander it! You've all heard that your body is a temple, so treat it accordingly. It's a precious gift that needs to be nurtured and cared for, not abused and forgotten.

When things take a turn for the worse and you suffer a major setback, financial or otherwise, your health may be all that you have to hang your optimistic hat on. My dad, when grappling with the many financial hardships we had to endure, would always say, "As long we have our health, there's always hope!" He was absolutely right on target, as per usual. When your health goes out the window, nothing else matters. Just as you can't buy happiness, all the money in the world can't buy your health, either. It won't be easy or convenient, but, to preserve or to improve your health, you must grab the bull by the horns and welcome the discomfort with open arms. It's for your own good—trust me: I'm a doctor (wink, wink)!

And there are few maladies that pose a greater risk to your health than heart disease or, more broadly speaking, cardio-vascular disease. Within the context of this broader clinical definition, *hypertension* (high blood pressure), *coronary artery disease* (heart-artery blockages), *stroke* (bleeding in the brain or clots lodged within it), *atrial fibrillation* (fast and irregular heart rhythm), and *heart failure* (a weak heart that can't deliver sufficient blood flow to the rest of the body) are the primary culprits on this ruthless death squad. All told, cardiovascular disease is the number one cause of death in the United States., accounting for one-third of all deaths, nearly 1 million deaths every year, and one death every minute! [*Centers for Disease Control* 2016 Statistics] So to say cardiovascular disease is an epidemic is a vast understatement, when you consider these sobering and somewhat terrifying statistics. The reality is that most of us are going to die from heart disease.

Looking solely at heart failure, which is where the bulk of my clinical efforts are focused, you'd be surprised to learn that it impacts nearly 3 percent of the entire population.

That's approximately 6 million people, with a prevalence that is expected to balloon to nearly 10 million by 2030. One in five adults develops heart failure, placing your lifetime risk at 20 percent. Unfortunately, however, heart failure doesn't command the same level of attention or consternation that other deadly diseases, like cancer, has garnered within the lay public. It's often too little too late when heart failure finally prompts undivided medical attention.

To put it in perspective, allow me to share the typical clinical scenario I encounter on an almost weekly basis. Much of what follows also appears in a recent blog I wrote on www. KevinMD.com, entitled, "It's Time We Approach Heart Failure like Cancer": I'm called to evaluate Mr. Smith, a fictional patient in his sixties with a known history of heart failure who's been admitted to the hospital with worsening shortness of breath. He's decompensated very precipitously at the point where I enter the picture, and things are not looking good. We've come a long way in heart surgery, but "resurrection" surgery is still not in our purview. I wish it were, but as I learned a while back from some the preeminent surgeons of our time, "Some hearts are so broken, even you can't fix them." This is one of those instances.

I'm forced to break the bad news: "I'm sorry, Mr. Smith. Your heart is very sick, and your body has irreversible damage. It's too dangerous to attempt a transplant or to implant a heart pump. There's nothing more we can do." And, just like that, we're forced to admit defeat and to relinquish yet another casualty in our lopsided battle with the heart failure epidemic. Off to hospice he goes...

Tragically, many of these patients present themselves long after being *followed closely* by their referring providers—"I've been seeing Mr. Smith in my office for years, and he's been pretty stable all along. He seemed fine just last week, so I'm not sure why he suddenly crashed."

Timing is everything. One month earlier, perhaps one year earlier, we may have had a fighting chance at saving Mr. Smith. It brings to mind some similarities with cancer, a curable disease if detected at an early stage and promptly treated. However, intentionally waiting until a cancer becomes metastatic before offering curative therapy would be unequivocally outlandish and indefensible.

Cancer is enviably very clear-cut that way. The moment a cancer is even suspected, be it a spot on a chest X-ray or a lump on a breast exam, a seek-and-destroy mission is reflexively launched. No questions asked. A flurry of activity ensues: scans, bloodwork, biopsies, and referral to a cancer specialist. No stone is left unturned. The train doesn't stop until the diagnosis is made and corresponding treatment is administered. If cancer is ruled out, well, then, it's back to the regularly scheduled programming. No harm, no foul.

Regretfully, this type of automated response does not exist in the heart failure world. For a disease with mortality rates surpassing many deadly cancers, the call to action when heart failure is diagnosed is comparatively subdued and haphazard. Medications with proven efficacy are prescribed and are titrated over time to maximally tolerated dosages. Absent overt deterioration, such as worsening heart failure symptoms or the need for hospitalization, this strategy of "guideline-directed medical therapy (GDMT)," as sanctioned by the American College of Cardiology (ACC), is the mainstay of heart failure management.

But GDMT has many nuances and pitfalls. Deciphering

whether a patient will tolerate any further increases in heart failure medications can baffle even the most seasoned clinician. And those tasked with making these tough calls include an array of family-medicine doctors, internists, and general cardiologists. With such divergent medical backgrounds, the adoption of ACC guidelines is by no means automatic. Many clinical studies have, in fact, documented inconsistent adherence to GDMT, with rates as disturbingly low as 20 percent.

For refractory heart failure, the guidelines recommend referral to a heart failure specialist, namely, a cardiologist subspecialized in *Advanced Heart Failure & Transplant Cardiology*, a subspecialty formally recognized barely a decade ago. On some level, it still lacks the street cred afforded other established medical specialties, a potential obstacle to timely referral. After all, many of these providers proudly proclaim they "know how to treat heart failure," and they may not see the necessity for referring their patient to a "specialist."

It's often only when things get out of hand that escalation of care is seriously contemplated. The horse is out of the barn, and now the only hope for salvage is a heart transplant or a mechanical heart pump. Our multidisciplinary "heart team" must conduct a thorough look under the hood, in search of any disqualifying findings. The incidental discovery of an occult cancer could, for example, derail the proceedings.

Of course, this evaluation would ideally occur electively as an outpatient, but many occur on a more urgent, inpatient basis. Furthermore, many of the patients surprisingly lack the basic prior testing we need to complete our assessment. Mammograms, colonoscopies, and other routine cancer screenings must now be rapidly orchestrated. This becomes logistically challenging, if not impossible, when time is of the essence and patients are critically ill. But we also can't afford the risk of unknowingly transplanting someone with an undiscovered cancer, only for it to spread uncontrollably after we start antirejection medications. Having to forego any of these tests may therefore eliminate heart transplant as a viable option.

Patients and their families are understandably very overwhelmed in these instances. They never saw this coming. Now, at the eleventh hour, they're grappling with the grim prospects of an imminently life-threatening illness. Again, we're left wondering—"If only they got to us sooner?" We all would have seen this coming and would have been prepared to meet the challenge.

To be clear, the referring providers are not at fault. These well-intentioned, fastidious clinicians are simply being duped by an unpredictable disease that doesn't play by the rules. It's the nature of the beast. Like a treated cancer that ominously recurs during supposed remission, so, too, can stable heart failure progress silently, without any discernible signs or symptoms. And when it eventually does become clinically obvious, it might very well be too late, as it was for Mr. Smith. Even within the confines of meticulously regulated clinical trials, up to a third of patients suffered progression in heart failure severity, while evading clinical detection. It's no wonder that, in real world practice, this stealth progression is even more widespread.

With nearly seven million people diagnosed, heart failure is a true national health crisis impacting all facets of medicine. To right the ship, we must all acknowledge heart failure for what it is, a moving target. The current paradigm is flawed, because it fails to account for that, relying too heavily on subjective interpretations of objective guidelines. Any diagnosis of heart failure should mandate a referral to a heart failure specialist, just as any cancer diagnosis warrants an automatic referral to an oncologist. This revised strategy would yield greater consistency and adherence to GDMT and would enable the early identification of patients that would benefit from advanced therapies, before decompensation. Patients and their families would be more prepared to meet these eventualities, having all requisite screening tests completed well in advance. The bottom line is that we would have more success stories and testimonials to share, rather than tragic lessons like those of Mr. Smith.

Okay, I'll get off my soapbox now, but I sincerely hope, for your sake, that the message sinks in—heart failure is deadly and vastly undertreated! Whatever you do, don't wait until it's too late! That's why, every chance I get, whether it's lecturing to medical students, speaking to colleagues in other specialties or to members of the community, or strategizing efforts with our marketing team, I make every effort to promote awareness of this deadly disease, encouraging an "earlier-rather-than-later" referral policy. Seeing these patients before irreversible complications occur can make all the difference in the world and can give us a fighting chance for victory.

Knowledge is power, and now that you're informed, you're also empowered to avoid becoming another statistic in the heart failure conflict. But, speaking more broadly on heart disease in general, I am often asked about what preventative strategies can be used to stave off this deadly illness, far and away the number one killer of our time. Luckily, the American Heart Association, with its "Life's Simple 7®" campaign, has laid out a set of readily achievable measures you can take to minimize your risk of developing heart disease. To learn more about the specifics of this program, I'd encourage you to visit their website at www.heart.org/en/healthy-living/healthy-lifestyle/my-life-check--lifes-simple-7.

American Heart Association's Life's Simple 7®		
1	Manage Blood Pressure	Getting at or under 120 / 80 is the goal and could likely entail anti-hypertensive medications being prescribed by your doctor, such as beta-blockers and ACE-inhibitors.
2	Control Cholesterol	A low-fat diet is key, but this may also be something for which your doctor may need to prescribe a cholesterol-lowering agent, usually a "statin" of some kind.
3	Reduce Blood Sugar	Also primarily manageable with a heart-healthy diet and staying in a healthy weight range. Medications may also be required to keep your sugar levels under control.
4	Get Active	At least moderate physical activity for a minimum of thirty minutes on most days of the week should do the trick.
5	Eat Better	A "heart-healthy" diet is low in fat, salt (sodium), with controlled portion size and lots of veggies.
6	Lose Weight	Getting to your ideal body weight will work wonders for your blood pressure, cholesterol levels, and blood sugars.
7	Stop Smoking	No exceptions, including vaping! All tobacco products are toxic to your cardiovascular system.

As you can see above, leading a heart-healthy lifestyle is not rocket science, and it definitely ain't heart surgery. They're largely self-explanatory, but I'd like to highlight a few points related to these measures. It should go without saying that all of us, at a minimum, should be getting an annual checkup with our primary-care doctor. For measures one through three, diet and exercise are undoubtedly helpful, but prescribed medications may still be necessary to keep your blood pressure, cholesterol, and sugar levels in check. Again, all the more reason you should be regularly seen by your physician—when in doubt, it's always a good idea to keep your doctor in the loop. Both of my parents paid the ultimate price for waiting until it was too late to seek medical care. But they didn't know any better, and you can't use that excuse! Without exception, you should be seen by a physician before embarking on any exercise or diet plan. Finally, I can't overemphasize how detrimental tobacco is to your health. It's a tough habit to kick, but arguably one of the most impactful steps you can take to prevent cancer, heart disease, and an untimely death!

The real take-home message here is that Life's Simple 7 are basic measures you or anybody else can take to reduce your risk of cardiovascular disease. It may not be the intense regimen of an elite athlete, but it will require concerted effort, discipline, willpower, and sacrifice on your part. Just as with *the Heart Way* of life, you can't become the best possible version of yourself unless you willingly subject yourself to some discomfort—no pain, no gain. Whether we're talking about basic health or being successful chasing your American Dream, you must accept discomfort as a fact of life. If it's too good to be true, like a new diet fad or a miracle pill that allows you to eat whatever you want but lose weight anyway, it usually is—don't kid yourself! Wanting the easy way out engenders the gullibility that drug and supplement companies are counting on to rake in the big profits. Don't fall for their traps! Basic heart-health maintenance is not a passive process. You need to be proactive and to take responsibility for your own well-being. Don't get complacent with your health!

Breaking old habits is no piece of cake. Sometimes it's less daunting to incorporate small changes or to start with just a couple of the Simple 7 initiatives to get the ball rolling. Almost no one can ever hit all 7 anyway, so don't get discouraged if you flounder a bit here and there—just keep at it! The important thing to remember is that taking one step is better than not taking any steps at all. Anytime you can enlist help from a professional, whether it's a dietician or a trainer, you'll have more accountability and encouragement. If dieticians and trainers are out of your price range, then enlist the help of a friend or a family member—hold each other accountable.

I've found that, in order to adhere to any diet or exercise plan, I have to plan ahead. This is where a lot of people fall short, myself included. If you're busy at work or at school all day, you may likely be ravenously hungry when lunchtime or dinner time rolls around. If you neglected to plan ahead or to pack your own healthy meal, just winging it at the cafeteria is a surefire recipe for failure. Just like shopping at the supermarket on an empty stomach, you're prone, in these instances, to make bad food choices, both in terms of quality and quantity, i.e., portion size. During surgical training, I'd have about twenty minutes between cases to eat, so I'd swoop into our hospital cafeteria, grab whatever was readily accessible, and inhale it! No time to wait in line at the healthy salad station. Why bother when the burgers, fries, and pizza were all conveniently packaged and ready for pickup—that's how they get you! Multiply that by ten years, and you can begin to understand how I managed to get about thirty pounds overweight!

To prevent this self-sabotage, what completely revolutionized my diet plan was meal prep—having my meals for the week already prepared in individual tupperware containers. The whole meal-prep craze had its origins in the professional bodybuilding world, where these musclebound freaks of nature must micromanage their dietary intake as if it's their job.

For me, meal prep was a true life hack that allowed me to get a real handle on portion size, while simultaneously adhering to body-friendly nutritive content. If eating were an Olympic sport, I'm confident that I'd be a world-class contender. I can put away a serious amount of food at quite the clip. Meal prep worked like a charm, as the ideal stopgap for my voracious appetite, and I benefited tremendously. Take the guessing out of food choices and stick to the program.

I've also found that it's easier to stick to this regimen if you allot yourself a "cheat day," when you let yourself go a bit and splurge on some unhealthy choices. Why cheat at all? When you're adopting dietary and lifestyle changes, it can be difficult to go cold turkey, so you're more likely to stay sane and keep at it, if you allow yourself the occasional treat. Just don't overdo it, and be sure to get right back on track with your plan!

But diet alone won't suffice to keep your heart health on the straight and narrow. Regular exercise must also become a priority. According to Life's Simple 7, "Adults should get a weekly total of at least 150 minutes of moderate aerobic activity or 75 minutes of vigorous aerobic activity or a combination of both, spread throughout the week."—How you do it is up to you.

Regular exercise doesn't have to be fancy or expensive; nor does it need to take place at a trendy gym with extravagant locker rooms. Even brisk walking counts. Whatever it is that floats your boat and keeps you coming back for more, just do it! Keep doing it, but look to make progress over time, in terms of "time, distance, or effort" (Life's Simple 7 website).

For me, the gym is my preferred haven to exercise, and weightlifting still holds a special place in my heart. Part of me is still that "gym rat" from high school, always up for "throwing some plates around" (meathead speak for powerlifting) in the weight room. It was always a great way for me to let off some steam and to decompress. However, I've learned of late that those glory days are long gone and that if I valued the structural integrity of my joints or my surgical livelihood, I needed to look beyond the heavy weight racks. I can't afford to have throbbing aches in my shoulders or lower back because I decided to go heavy on bench presses or dead lifts. Besides, doing my same old scripted workouts from circa 1992 was not working for me anymore. I wasn't seen any gains. To start seeing some progress, I had to completely change up the routine and begrudgingly incorporate much more aerobic exercise, like running on a treadmill.

Having never been a big fan of long-distance running, I absolutely hated these changes at first. Running, for me, was supposed to be explosive bursts of speed, with an objective in mind, like tackling the opposing team's ball carrier on the football field. A few years ago, when I first began implementing these changes, I could barely run for five minutes on a treadmill before completely running out of steam. I was miserably out of shape. But rather than giving up or finding an alternate form of cardio, I decided to dig in my heels and to keep grinding. The plan was simple: each time I'd hop on the treadmill, I'd push myself to do better than the last time by running at a faster pace or for a longer duration of time. I was competing against just myself. As time went on, I found myself looking forward to the day's run and to the challenge it presented.

The incremental progress I was steadily making began to be noticeable in my physique and was reflected on the weighing scale. I lost a ton of weight and felt like I was in the best shape of my life. Am I pleased and satisfied? I'm pleased, but I'm definitely not satisfied. I will continue to push myself. I'm still not ready for prime time, but I intend to eventually be marathon- or ironman-ready. Getting there will be a grueling process, but I'm looking forward to it. I'm up for the challenge.

You see, it's never too late to turn over a new leaf and to change for the better. Health and success are not guarantees. Neither is the American Dream. They are all conditional, one and the same. For those daring and willing, it's open season on all of the above! Modern society, with its innumerable diversions and self-serving agendas, has most of its disillusioned and misguided followers believing otherwise. But the fact is that there are no winners and losers in this life. There are those that *choose* to chase victory and to live life on their terms, and there are those that don't. The latter succumb to the status quo and never try to rekindle their extinguished hopes and dreams. They're content with the safety and certainty afforded by just sitting out the race.

We all have free will, and we all have a choice. You can choose to live aimlessly, halfheartedly going with the flow and suppressing that inner voice, the one beckoning you to unleash your full potential and to grab the world by storm. In your reading this book, I hope to count you among those that choose, instead, to heed that inner voice. You see clear through all the hype, the smoke, and the mirrors. You're not buying what most of society is selling. You haven't lost your hope or your nerve. And that's because you know that when there's a will, there's a way—*the Heart Way,* to be exact!

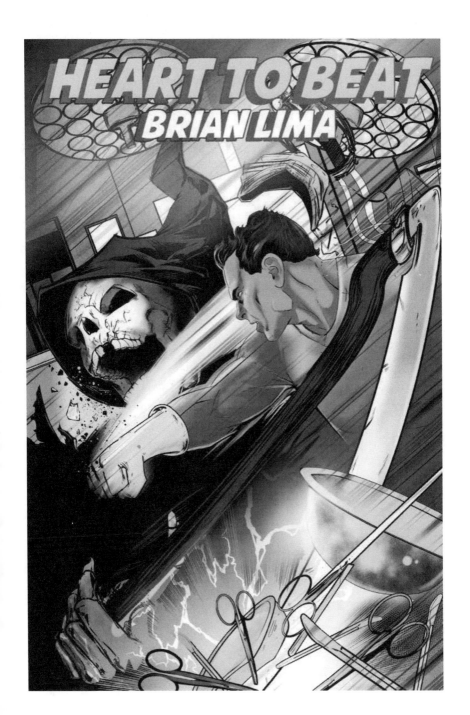

ABOUT THE AUTHOR

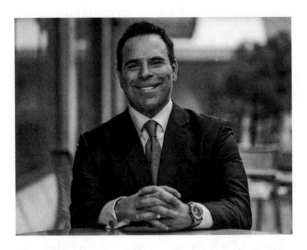

Dr. Brian Lima is an author, a husband, and a surgeon who built a reputation as a renowned cardiac surgeon at Baylor University Medical Center (BUMC) in Dallas, Texas. He was recruited to North Shore University Hospital (Northwell Health) in 2017 to lead the first and only heart-transplant program on Long Island, and he was appointed Associate Professor of Surgery. Dr. Lima was previously the Surgical Director of Mechanical Circulatory Support at BUMC, where he also served as Director of Clinical Research in Cardiac Transplantation and Mechanical Circulatory Support. Dr. Lima was one of the primary cardiac-transplant surgeons at BUMC and was instrumental in building one of the busiest heart-transplant centers in the country—including the nation's lowest waiting list times.

Dr. Lima is a recognized authority on surgical therapies for advanced heart failure, having published nearly eighty articles in peer-reviewed journals and numerous book chapters; he has also presented at several national and international conferences. In addition to heart transplantation, Dr. Lima's expertise encompasses the entire spectrum of adult cardiac surgery and the surgical management of heart failure with mechanical-support devices.

Originally from Kearny, New Jersey, Dr. Lima attended Cornell University for his undergraduate studies as a Cornell National Scholar, graduating magna cum laude in Chemistry. Dr. Lima attended medical school at Duke University School of Medicine, receiving a Dean's Full Tuition Scholarship and graduating with Alpha Omega Alpha distinction. During medical school, Dr. Lima was a recipient of the prestigious Stanley J. Sarnoff Research Fellowship Award in cardiovascular sciences, which funded a year of investigation at the Transplantation Biology Research Center of the Massachusetts General Hospital/Harvard Medical School. Following his general-surgery residency training at Duke University Medical Center, Dr. Lima completed his formal heart-surgery training at the Cleveland Clinic, where he received the Dr. Charles H. Bryan Annual Clinical Excellence Award in Cardiovascular Surgery.